Revitalize

Ultimate Guide To The World Of Diet And Nutrition For A Vibrant Life

By
Dr. Rachel Boston

Table of content

Introduction

Diet refers to a specific eating plan followed for health or weight management purposes. Diet, in a broader sense, refers to the overall pattern of eating habits and choices that someone follows. It includes the types of food consumed, portion sizes, meal timings, and salutary preferences. It can be an important part of keeping a healthy body. Another aspect of diet is that it can be customized based on individual requirements and pretensions. Some people follow specific diets like vegetarian, vegan, paleo, or keto, while others concentrate on portion control or calorie counting. It is essential to find a style of diet that works for you, and each is about nourishing your body and enjoying the food you eat. Continuing on the content of diet, it's important to prioritize nutrient-dense foods like fruits, vegetables, whole grains, spare proteins, and healthy fats. These provide essential vitamins, minerals, and energy for our bodies. It's also good to stay doused and limit the input of reused foods and added sugars. Remember: small changes over time can lead to big advancements in your overall health and well-being. Let's dive deeper into diet and nutrition. Did you know that a well-balanced diet can have multitudinous benefits? It can support healthy weight operations, boost energy situations, strengthen the vulnerable system, and reduce the threat of habitual conditions. Plus, certain nutrients, like omega-3 adipose acids set up in fish, can support brain health. It's fascinating how the food we eat can have such a profound impact on our overall well-being. Did you also know that different foods have different effects on our bodies? For example, fruits and vegetables are packed with vitamins and minerals that help keep us healthy and strong. On the other hand, reused foods high in added sugars and unhealthy fats can have negative effects on our health. It's all about achieving balance and making choices that nourish our bodies and make us feel good inside and out.

A diet goes beyond just what we eat. It also encompasses our eating habits, portion sizes, meal timing, and indeed, our relationship with food. It's about being aware of our choices, practicing temperance, and listening to our body's hunger and wholeness cues. Also, factors like physical exertion, stressful situations, and sleep patterns can impact how our bodies process and use the nutrients in our diet. It's about espousing a healthy life that includes regular exercise, proper hydration, and acceptable sleep. Physical exertion helps to strengthen our muscles, ameliorate cardiovascular health, and boost our mood. Hydration is important for digestion, rotation, and overall fleshly functions. And getting enough quality sleep allows our bodies to repair and recharge. So, a well-rounded approach to health involves more than just what is on our plates. More on the factors that help impact our health:Regular exercise not only helps to keep our bodies fit, but it also releases endorphins that boost our mood and reduce stress. Whether it's going for a run, dancing, or playing a sport, the conditioning that you enjoy can make exercise more delightful and sustainable. Hydration is essential for maintaining optimal fleshly functions, perfecting digestion, and keeping our skin healthy. And getting enough quality sleep allows our bodies to repair, recharge, and support overall cognitive function. So, remember to move, drink water, and catch those Z's for a well-rounded, healthy life.

A healthy diet consists of a variety of different factors. It's important to include fruits and vegetables for essential vitamins and minerals. Whole grains give fiber and energy. Spare proteins, such as chicken, fish, and beans, are important for muscle growth and form. Healthy fats, like those found in avocados and nuts, are vital for brain function.

 Let's expand on each element of a healthy diet. Fruits and vegetables are packed with essential vitamins and minerals that keep our bodies performing well. They provide a wide range of nutrients and antioxidants that support our vulnerable systems and overall health. Incorporating a variety of various fruits and veggies into our diets is a great way to ensure we are getting a good blend of nutrients. Whole grains, like oats, brown rice, and whole wheat bread are an amazing source of strength and fiber. They help keep us feeling full and satisfied, regulate our digestion, and give us a steady release of energy throughout the day. Including whole grains in our diet can also help reduce the threat of certain habitual conditions. Spare proteins, such as chicken, fish, tofu, and beans, are essential for muscle growth and form. They give us important amino acids that our bodies need to make and maintain strong muscles. Including a variety of spare proteins in our diets ensures we are getting a good balance of nutrients. Healthy fats, like those found in avocados, nuts, and olive oil, are important for brain function and overall health. They provide us with essential adipose acids that our bodies cannot produce on their own. Incorporating these healthy fats into our diet can help ameliorate cognitive function and support heart health. Incipiently, staying doused with water is pivotal for our overall well-being. Water helps regulate our body temperature, aids in digestion, and supports healthy skin. It's important to drink water throughout the day to stay hydrated and keep our bodies performing optimally. A healthy diet is all about balance and temperance. Incorporating these different factors into our diets can help us achieve a well-rounded and nutritional diet.

Nutrition is all about the study of how food nourishes our bodies and the process of carrying and exercising the nutrients from the food we eat. It's about understanding the significance of different nutrients like vitamins, minerals, carbohydrates, proteins, and fats and how they contribute to our overall health and well-being.

Nutrition helps us make informed choices about what we eat to support our bodies' requirements and maintain optimal health. Embrace the power of nutrition and energy in our bodies for a vibrant and healthy life. The collaboration of a balanced diet and nutrition is like a dynamic brace! A balanced diet ensures that you are getting all the necessary nutrients your body needs, while nutrition focuses on the wisdom behind those nutrients and how they impact your health. When you combine the two, you are nourishing your body with the right foods in the right quantities, promoting optimal health and well-being. It's all about changing that sweet spot where you are enjoying a variety of nutrient-dense foods while still allowing yourself some flexibility and enjoyment.

Macronutrients relate to the three main factors of our diet: carbohydrates, proteins, and fats. Carbohydrates give us energy, proteins help with muscle growth and form, and fats give essential nutrients and support colorful functions in our bodies. It's important to have a balanced input of these macronutrients to support our overall health and well-being. Carbohydrates are the body's main root of strength. They're broken down into glucose, which energizes our cells and provides energy for diurnal conditioning. Complex carbs, like whole grains and vegetables, are digested more slowly and give sustained energy, while simple carbs, like sticky foods, give a quick energy boost.

Proteins are pivotal for structure and repair, similar to muscles, organs, and cells. They're made up of amino acids, which are the structural blocks of proteins. Animal sources like meat, flesh, and dairy provide complete proteins with all essential amino acids, while factory-ground sources like legumes, tofu, and quinoa can be combined to get all the necessary amino acids. .

Fats play a variety of roles in our bodies. They give energy, help absorb fat-responsive vitamins(A, D, E, and K), and are essential for the production of hormones. Unsaturated fats, found in avocados, nuts, and olive oil, are healthier options that can support heart health. Saturated and trans fats, set up in fried foods and reused snacks, should be limited as they can increase the threat of heart disease.

Reminder: It's important to have a balanced input of macronutrients to support overall health. Each macronutrient has its own unique benefits, so incorporating a variety of foods is crucial. Micronutrients relate to the essential vitamins and minerals that our bodies need in lower quantities. They play a pivotal role in colorful fleshly functions, similar to supporting vulnerable functions, maintaining healthy bones, and assisting in energy production. Examples of micronutrients include vitamins like vitamin C and vitamin D and minerals like iron, calcium, and zinc. It's important to have a balanced diet that includes a variety of foods to ensure we get an acceptable input of these micronutrients. They're essential vitamins and minerals that our bodies need in lower amounts to support colorful functions. These nutrients are necessary for maintaining good health. For instance, vitamins such as vitamin C help boost our vulnerable system and promote healthy skin, while minerals like iron are necessary for proper oxygen transport in the body.

Including a different range of foods in our diet, such as fruits, vegetables, whole grains, and spare proteins, can help ensure an acceptable input of these micronutrients. Salutary guidelines are recommendations that give guidance on what and how much we should eat to maintain good health. They offer advice on colorful aspects of our diet, such as the types and quantities of food to consume as well as healthy eating patterns. These guidelines frequently emphasize the significance of consuming a variety of nutrient-rich foods, such as fruits, vegetables, whole grains, spare proteins, and healthy fats. They also punctuate the need to limit the input of added sugars, sodium, and saturated fats. Following salutary guidelines can help promote overall health and reduce the threat of habitual conditions. It's always a good idea to consult with a healthcare professional or listed dietitian for substantiated guidance grounded on your specific requirements and pretensions. They give us advice on all kinds of stuff, like what kinds of foods to eat and how to make sure we are getting enough of the good stuff. They are each about balance and temperance, encouraging us to eat a variety of foods from different food groups, like fruits, veggies, whole grains, spare proteins, and healthy fats. They also remind us to watch out for effects like added sugars, sodium, and unhealthy fats. By following these guidelines, we can ameliorate our overall health and reduce the threat of getting sick. But remember : everyone's different, so it's always a good idea to sputter with a healthcare professional or a registered dietitian to get substantiated advice that fits your requirements and pretensions. Oh, the impact of diet on health is huge! What we eat plays a major part in our overall well-being. A healthy diet can provide us with the essential nutrients our bodies need to function properly, support our vulnerable systems, and keep our energy levels up. It can also help maintain a healthy weight, reduce the threat of habitual conditions like heart disease and diabetes, and indeed ameliorate our mood and internal health. On the other hand, a poor diet, high in reused foods, added sugars, and unhealthy fats, can increase the threat of health problems and make us feel sluggish and bad. So, it's important to fuel our bodies with nutritional foods and make healthy choices to support our long-term health and vitality! A healthy diet can have a positive impact on our bodies in numerous ways.

Eating a balanced diet that includes a variety of fruits, vegetables, whole grains, spare proteins, and healthy fats provides us with essential vitamins, minerals, and antioxidants that support our vulnerable system and promote good health. It can also ameliorate our digestion, give us further energy, and indeed enhance our skin's appearance. On the other side, a poor diet high in reused foods, added sugars, and unhealthy fats can lead to weight gain, nutrient scarcity, and an increased threat of habitual conditions. So, by making smart food choices, we can nourish our bodies and enjoy a healthier, happier life. The diet plays a pivotal part in weight management! What we eat directly affects our weight. A balanced diet that includes nutrient-dense foods can help us maintain a healthy weight. By fasting on whole foods like fruits, vegetables, whole grains, spare proteins, and healthy fats, we can give our bodies the necessary nutrients while keeping our calorie input in check. These foods are frequently lower in calories and higher in fiber, which helps us feel full and satisfied. It's important to find a balance and make sustainable changes to our eating habits to support long-term weight loss. Remember : it's not just about confining calories but also nourishing our bodies with wholesome foods. By making nutritional food choices, we can take a visionary step towards preventing conditions and promoting long-term health.

There are many types of diets that people follow based on their preferences and health pretensions.

The Mediterranean diet, which emphasizes fruits, vegetables, whole grains, and healthy fats; the ketogenic diet, which is high in fats, moderate in protein, and veritably low in carbohydrates; the submissive diet, which excludes meat but includes plant-based foods; and the vegan diet, which excludes all beast products. Other diets include the paleo diet, the dash diet, and the flexitarian diet. It's important to find a diet that works stylishly for you and aligns with your health intentions and life. Let's dive into each diet one by one.

Mediterranean diet

This diet is inspired by the traditional eating habits of people in Mediterranean countries. It focuses on consuming a plenitude of fruits, vegetables, whole grains, legumes, nuts, seeds, and healthy fats like olive oil. It also includes moderate quantities of fish, flesh, and dairy products. Red meat and reused foods are limited. The Mediterranean diet has been associated with multitudinous health benefits, including a reduced threat of heart disease and better brain health.

Ketogenic diet

The ketogenic diet is a low-carbohydrate, high-fat diet that aims to switch the body's primary energy source from carbohydrates to fats. By drastically reducing carbohydrate input and adding fat consumption, the body enters a state called ketosis, where it burns fat for energy. This diet frequently includes foods like flesh, fish, eggs, avocados, nuts, and healthy canvases. It has gained popularity for weight loss and managing certain medical conditions like epilepsy, but it may not be suitable for everyone.

Vegetarian diet

The vegetarian diet excludes meat but includes factory-ground foods like fruits, vegetables, grains, legumes, nuts, and seeds. Some may also consume dairy products and eggs, while others avoid them. This diet provides essential nutrients while reducing the input of saturated fats and cholesterol set up in meat. Vegetarian diets have been associated with lower pitfalls of heart disease, high blood pressure, and certain cancers.

Vegan diet

The vegan diet takes vegetarianism a step further by banning all animal products, including meat, dairy, eggs, and honey. It focuses on factory-ground foods like fruits, vegetables, grains, legumes, nuts, and seeds. Vegans frequently choose this diet for ethical, environmental, or health reasons. With proper planning, a vegan diet can provide all the necessary nutrients, but attention should be paid to sources of protein, vitamin B12, iron, and omega-3 adipose acids. 5. Paleo diet

The Paleo diet is grounded in the idea of eating foods analogous to what our ancestors ate during the Paleolithic period. It emphasizes whole foods like spare flesh, fish, fruits, vegetables, nuts, and seeds while banning reused foods, grains, legumes, and dairy products. The thing is to consume foods

that our bodies are genetically acclimated to, promoting better digestion and overall health. Still, the paleo diet may be restrictive and may not provide all the necessary nutrients.
 Dash diet
 It stands for Dietary Approaches to Stop Hypertension. It's a diet specifically designed to help lower blood pressure.The dash diet emphasizes eating fruits, vegetables, whole grains, spare proteins, and low-fat dairy products. It also encourages reducing sodium input and limiting foods high in saturated fats and added sugars. It's a great option if you are looking to keep your blood pressure in check.
There are several benefits to following a healthy diet. Weight management:A balanced diet can help you maintain a healthy weight or indeed lose weight if demanded.
Advanced energy situations: Eating nutritional foods can give you the energy you need to stay active and focused throughout the day.
Reduced threat of habitual conditions:A healthy diet can lower the threat of developing conditions like heart disease, diabetes, and certain cancers.
More digestion: Eating a diet rich in fiber can promote healthy digestion and help with constipation.
Stronger, more vulnerable system: Nutrient-rich foods can support a strong, vulnerable system, helping you fight off illnesses and infections. Improved mood and internal health: Certain nutrients, like omega-3 adipose acids, have been linked to better mood and cognitive function.
Remember : It's important to find a diet that works for you and fits your life. It's all about making sustainable, long-term changes for your overall well-being. Making good food choices is pivotal for promoting health and well-being! The food we eat provides us with essential nutrients that our bodies need to function properly. A balanced diet rich in fruits, vegetables, whole grains, spare proteins, and healthy fats can provide the necessary vitamins, minerals, and antioxidants to support our vulnerable system, maintain a healthy weight, and reduce the

threat of habitual conditions. It can also ameliorate our energy situation, mood, and overall quality of life. So, choosing nutritional foods is a great way to take care of our bodies and promote our health. When it comes to promoting health and well-being, the significance of food choices cannot be overstated. The foods we choose to consume have a direct impact on our overall health.

Finally: nutrient-dense options like fruits, vegetables, whole grains, spare proteins, and healthy fats provide our bodies with the necessary vitamins, minerals, and antioxidants to function optimally. These nutrients support our vulnerable system, help maintain a healthy weight, and reduce the threat of habitual conditions such as heart disease, diabetes, and certain cancers. In addition, a balanced diet can enhance our energy situation, ameliorate our mood, and contribute to our overall vitality and quality of life. Nutrients play vital roles in supporting our health and wellbeing. They give us the energy our bodies need to function properly, helping us stay alive. Also, nutrients like vitamins and minerals support our vulnerable functions, helping us fight off illnesses and infections. They also play a pivotal role in maintaining the health of our organs, which they serve optimally.

Foundation Of Wellness : Building A Strong Health Routine

Power Of Diet: Fueling Your Health

A healthy diet is all about making good food choices that nourish your body. It includes eating a variety of fruits, vegetables, whole grains, lean proteins, and healthy fats. These foods provide essential nutrients like vitamins, minerals, and antioxidants that support your overall health. It's also important to stay doused by drinking plenty of water. Reminder; balance is crucial! enjoying treats in moderation is part of a healthy diet too. So let's keep it simple and concentrate on nourishing our bodies with succulent and nutritional foods.

Impact of nutrition on overall well-being

A good nutritive status is important for maintaining normal body function and precluding or mollifying the dysfunction caused by mental or external factors. Nutritional scarcity frequently affects disabled function, and, again, inputs in recommended levels can renew or further enhance body functions. An increasing number of studies are revealing that diet and nutrition are critical not only for physiology and body composition but also have significant effects on mood and mental well-being. In particular, western dietary habits have been the object of several research studies focused on the relationship between nutrition and mental health. This review aims to epitomize the current knowledge about the relationship between the input of specific micro- and macronutrients, including eicosapentaenoic acid, docosahexaenoic acid, nascent tocopherol, magnesium, and folic acid, and mental health, with particular reference to their dietary effects on stress, sleep diseases, anxiety, and mild cognitive impairment, as well as neuropsychiatric diseases, all significantly affecting the quality of life of an increasing number of people. Overall data support a positive role for the nutrients mentioned above in the preservation of normal brain function and mental well-being, also through the control of neuroinflammation, and encourage their integration into a well-balanced and varied diet accompanied by a healthy life. This strategy is of particular significance when considering global mortality and the fact that the brain suffers significantly from the life-long impact of stress factors. Nutrition is an important factor in relation to the well-being of a person. Nutrition is related to better child, child, and motherly health, stronger immune systems, safer gestation and parturition, a lower risk of non-communicable conditions(such as diabetes and cardiovascular diseases), and life.

Nutrition and Well-being

We're all apprehensive of the benefits of good nutrition and physical health. It improves heart health and reduces the risk of diabetes, high blood pressure, and certain cancers, but what about taking care of the mind? Do those redundant chocolate bars and the lack of vegetables in your diet have an influence on your mood? The simple answer is yes; they can have a massive impact on your mental health. Recent substantiation suggests that good nutrition is essential for our mental health and that several mental health conditions may be caused by dietary factors. nutrition tends to be the most egregious yet under-recognized factor in the development of major trends in mental health. Still, the body of substantiation linking diet and mental health is growing at a rapid-fire pace. As well as its impact on short- and long-term mental health, much of the research indicates that food plays an important part in the development, management, and prevention of specific mental health problems such as cavity, schizophrenia, attention deficit hyperactivity diseases , and Alzheimer's diseases . Along with exercise, quality sleep, and stress management, getting the right balance of nutrients in your diet can go a long way towards balancing your mood and anxiety situations. Your brain is always" on, indeed, when you're asleep. Although the brain accounts for only 2 percent of the weight of the body, it uses up 20 percent of the energy that's deduced from the food we eat far more than any other organ. This means that your brain requires a constant force of energy. that energy comes from the foods you eat, and what's in that energy makes all the difference. This starts with eating nutritionally balanced diets. In every meal, it's important that you include a portion of protein along with complex carbohydrates and a variety of vegetables. Protein, including protein-rich foods at mealtime, is veritably important because protein contains the amino acid tryptophan, which is the structure block for the serotonin product, a brain chemical that promotes a feeling of well-being. Complex carbohydrates are inversely important. Complex carbs give us a slow, steady release of energy and encourage a slow, steady release of serotonin. so, they've got a long-lasting positive effect on our energy and mood. Vitamins B6, B12, and omega-3 fatty acids impact serotonin, which, as preliminarily mentioned, is necessary for mood regulation. A good amount of people are well aware of the benefits that eating a balanced diet has on their physical health, but do you know how it benefits our mental health? Further and further research is coming to light on the impact food has on both our overall mental health and specific mental ailments like depression and anxiety.

The relationship between food and mood

Let's take a closer look at how food and mood are related and what part our gut health plays. Eating a diet that's well-rounded and nutrient-rich can help to improve mood, increase energy levels, and help you feel better easily. There are several at play then, from the number of carbohydrates you eat to the way scarcity of vitamins and minerals affects mental health.

Carbohydrates and eating regularly

In order for your brain to be suitable to concentrate, It needs energy(20% of all energy demanded by the body is used by the brain). When we don't have enough energy for the brain, we can feel weak, tired, and unfit to think easily. eating regular meals containing some carbohydrates will help with this. Alongside starchy foods like pasta and rice, sources of carbohydrates include wholegrains, fruits, vegetables, and legumes. lower-fat dairy

When your blood glucose rises and falls rapidly, it can have an impact on your mood, making you feel perverse and low and indeed driving symptoms of anxiety. Keeping your blood glucose levels steady throughout the day is crucial. try foods that release energy slowly, like oats, cereals, nuts, and seeds, and aim to eat smaller portions spaced out throughout the day. proteins and fats alongside the energy it gets from carbohydrates, your brain needs amino acids to help regulate studies and feelings .

As protein contains amino acids, it's important to get enough of this in your diet. Protein is set up in lean meat, fish, eggs, nuts and seeds, soy products, and legumes. Some people may be under the impression that all fat is bad for us, but this isn't the case.

Fatty acids, like omega-3 and omega-6, are essential for our minds to think well. Healthy fats can be found in nuts, seeds, oily fish, poultry, avocados, dairy products, and eggs. Our focus on low-fat diets may have also inadvertently affected our mental well-being. The brain is around 60 percent fat, and omega-3 fatty acids are important for neurons to communicate effectively. Vitamins and minerals : When we don't get enough of certain vitamins and minerals, both our physical and mental health can suffer. The best way to ensure you're getting enough of the vitamins and minerals you need is to eat a varied and balanced diet rich in fruit and vegetables.

 Iron : A lack of iron can lead you to feel weak, tired, and sleepy. Foods rich in iron include red meat, poultry , fish, beans, and fortified cereals.

 Vitamin B: Not getting enough b1, b3, and b12 can make you feel low, tired, and perverse. Animal protein foods, such as meat, fish, eggs, dairy, and fortified cereals, are rich in b vitamins.

Folate : When you don't get enough folate, you can be at risk of feeling depressed. Folate can be found in green vegetables, citrus fruits, liver, beans, and fortified foods like marmite.

 Selenium : Selenium insufficiency may increase the chance of feeling depressed and other negative moods. Good sources of selenium include brazil nuts, seeds, and wholemeal bread, meat, and fish. A helpful way to make sure your diet is nutrient-rich is to make sure you're getting at least five portions of fruit and vegetables every day.

Dehydration anxiety : Hydration and nutrition go hand in hand, but the vast quantum of information available can frequently overwhelm us and bring feelings of anxiety. For some, these feelings can be severe. Dehydration anxiety is a fear that you aren't drinking acceptable quantities of water. You may sweat going anywhere without your water bottle. This fear can lead to a higher consumption of water than your body requires which can lead to illness. The fear stems from not giving your body sufficient hydration to perform at its best. This habitual form of anxiety is nearly linked to compulsive-obsessive diseases and orthorexia. Signs of dehydration anxiety include: feeling a sense of dread when you don't have your water bottle; fussing about where to get water from,e.g., when shopping or traveling; passing fear attacks when water isn't incontinently available.

Nutritional Remedies And Hydration

The recommended six to eight spectacles of water per day (roughly two liters) can be used as a general guideline for your water input, alongside consideration of your individual dietary requirements. The specific amount of hydration demanded varies from person to person, so it's important to tune into your whole life when considering how important water is to provide sufficient hydration for you. Nutrition therapist Karen Alexander says that it's not only the water you drink; your diet, gender, age, exercise, and life are also contributing factors to your water requirements.However, you'll need to drink further to ensure you're getting enough if your input of vegetables and fruit is low.

Gut Health and Mental Health

The link between our gut health and our mental health is getting clearer. Frequently dubbed the second brain', our digestive system produces over 90 percent of all serotonin(the happy hormone) in our body. Our gut can also affect impunity and adaptability to stress, which can both have an effect on our mood. Having a healthy digestive system, in general, ensures we're able to absorb the vitamins, minerals, and nutrients our bodies need to thrive. Frequently, when we're feeling stressed out or anxious, we'll feel it in our gut. Digestion may speed up or decelerate, depending on how we're feeling. to keep your gut happy, ensure you eat plenty of fiber, get lots of fluid, and do regular exercise.

Fermented foods help in giving the bacteria that are good for our energy, nutrition, and immune system functions. Our immune system is a network of pathways that help cover our body against dangerous microbes, conditions, bacteria, sponges, and contagions. There are two main parts in the immune system. The first is the innate immune system that we're born with, which creates a physical and chemical barrier to cover the body from dangerous raiders. Examples include the skin, mucous membranes, stomach acid, enzymes that make antibacterial composites, and the blood-brain barrier. The alternative is the acquired, or adaptive, immune system. It develops when exposed to raiders. It helps your body produce antibodies to fight off those raiders. It also changes and adapts throughout our lives to protect us from dangerous conditions. Also, if the raiders strike again, the acquired immune system will remember the foreign substance and fight it off hastily.

 Likewise, numerous factors can affect your immune system, including exercise, sleep, stress situations, alcohol consumption, and weight. I want to concentrate on diet and nutrition.

So, let's take a closer look at the role they play in supporting the function of your body's immune system.

- Balancing your gut and your plate : A balanced diet helps your cells and organs function while keeping your body healthy. The gut is a significant point for antimicrobial products and immune responses. What you eat can impact your gut's microbiome, determining what microbes live in your intestines. Your body and immune system bear micronutrients(vitamins and minerals) to serve you completely. For this reason, a healthy diet rich in fruits, vegetables, whole grains, legumes, protein, dairy, and water is essential. Erecting a healthy plate at every meal can be a great place to start. Try choosing water or milk as your libation. Also, concentrate on filling half of your plate with vegetables and fruits; add in protein, whole grains, and healthy fat. Reminder : Processed , high-fat, and sugary foods or potables should be limited and only consumed in moderation.

- Maximizing your micronutrients : Your diet must include several vital micronutrients for your immune cells to grow and serve properly. Six essential micronutrients to boost your immune functions include: Iron - Allows cells to develop and gain sources of iron can include red meat, leafy greens , beans, nuts, and fortified cereals. Vitamin C - This helps stimulate the conformation of antibodies as well as the production and function of white blood cells. Some sources of vitamin C are bell peppers, tomatoes, broccoli and oranges. Vitamin A - This nutrient helps protect against infections and is an anti-inflammatory vitamin that enhances immune function. Sources of vitamin A include leafy green vegetables, tomatoes, cantaloupe, milk, eggs, and fish canvases. Vitamin D regulates antimicrobial proteins that help kill pathogens in your body. Sources of vitamin D can include fortified dairy, salmon, egg yolk, tuna fish, and beef liver. Vitamin E - This is an antioxidant and helps cover the integrity of the cell membrane, preventing damage from free radicals. Sources of vitamin E include wheat, sunflower seeds, peanut adulation, pumpkin, bell peppers, and leafy greens. Zinc - this micronutrient helps support the immune response and is vital for crack repair. Sources of zinc include milk, nuts, poultry , seeds, whole grains, and poultry.also, a factory-rich diet high in fiber and containing prebiotics and probiotics can help support the growth of microbes, increase immune cell exertion, and help your body fight infections. Probiotic foods that contain beneficial live bacteria that help improve digestive health include yogurt, kefir, kombucha tea, buttermilk, and fermented vegetables such as tempeh, kimchi, and sauerkraut.

- Strive for variety : Diets low in variety can negatively affect a person's immune system and cause nutritional scarcity. It can be particularly challenging for some people to acquire nutrient-dense foods, especially those with increased nutrient requirements. For example, groups at risk of developing nutrient scarcity can include food insecure homes, individuals with restrictive diets, the elderly, critically ill cases, pregnant and lactating women, babies, and children. In most cases, these populations can condense with a vitamin and mineral authority to help fill any nutritive gaps and scarcities. Still, you should consult a health care provider before adding new supplements to your routine.
- Significance of fruits and vegetables in a diet :
  Vegetables and fruit basket of food, including grapes, apples, asparagus, onions, lettuce, carrots, melon, and bananas corn . Vegetables and fruits are an important part of a healthy diet, and variety is as important as volume. eat aplenty every day. A diet rich in vegetables and fruits can lower blood pressure, reduce the risk of heart disease and stroke, help some types of cancer, lower the risk of eye and digestive problems, and have a positive impact on maintaining your blood sugar, which can help keep your appetite in check. Eating non-starchy vegetables and fruits like apples, pears, and green, leafy vegetables may indeed promote weight loss. Their low glycemic loads help blood sugar levels, which can increase hunger. at least nine different families of fruits and vegetables live, each with potentially hundreds of different factory composites that are dietary health. This not only ensures a greater diversity of dietary factory chemicals but also creates eye-appealing reproductions.

Tips to eat more vegetables and fruits each day

Keep your fruits where you can see it. Place several ready-to-eat, washed whole fruits in a coliseum or store diced various fruits in a glass bowl in the refrigerator to tempt a sweet tooth.
 On most days, try to get at least one serving from each of the following orders: dark green leafy vegetables; orange fruits and vegetables; red fruits and vegetables; legumes(beans) and peas; and citrus fruits.
Choose other vegetables that are packed with different nutrients and slowly digested carbohydrates. Make it a meal,try cooking new recipes that include more vegetables. salads, and stir-feasts are just a few ideas for adding a number of delicious vegetables to your recipes. vegetables, fruits, and cardiovascular diseases.
 There's compelling evidence that a diet rich in fruits and vegetables can lower the risk of heart disease and stroke.
 A meta-analysis of cohort studies following 469,551 people found that an advanced input of fruits and vegetables is associated with a reduced risk of death from cardiovascular diseases , with an average reduction in risk of 4 for each fresh serving per day of fruit and vegetables. The largest and longest study to date, done as part of the harvard-grounded nurses' health study and health professional follow-up study, included nearly 110,000 men and women whose health and dietary habits were followed 14 times. The higher the average diurnal input of fruits and vegetables, the lower the chance of developing a cardiovascular problem. Compared with those in the smallest order of fruit and vegetable input(lower than 1.5 servings a day), those who equaled 8 or more servings a day were 30 times less likely to have had a heart attack or stroke. Although all fruits and vegetables likely contributed to this benefit, green, leafy vegetables, such as lettuce, spinach, and mustard leafs were most explosively associated with a dropped risk of cardiovascular diseases. Yellow vegetables such as broccoli, cauliflower, cabbage, brussels sprouts, bok choy, and kale; and citrus fruits such as oranges, limes, and grapefruit also made important contributions. When experimenters combined findings from the harvard studies with several other

long-term studies in the U.S and Europe looked at coronary heart complaint and stroke independently, they set up an analogous defensive effect: individuals who ate more than 5 servings of fruits and vegetables per day had roughly a 20 percent lower risk of coronary heart complaint and stroke compared with individuals who ate less than 3 servings per day. Blood pressure - The Dietary Approaches To Stop Hypertension(DASH) study examined the effect on blood pressure of a diet that was rich in fruits, vegetables, and low-fat dairy products and that confined the quantity of saturated and total fat. The experimenters found that people with high blood pressure who followed this diet reduced their systolic blood pressure(the upper number of a blood pressure reading) by about 11 mm hg and their diastolic blood pressure(the lower number) by nearly 6 mm hg—as much as specifics can achieve. A randomized trial known as the optimal macronutrient intake trial for heart health(omniheart) showed that this fruit and vegetable-rich diet lowered blood pressure indeed more when some of the carbohydrate was replaced with healthy unsaturated fat or protein. In 2014, a meta-analysis of clinical trials and experimental studies found that consumption of a vegetarian diet was associated with lower blood pressure. Cancer - Multitudinous early studies revealed what appeared to be a strong link between eating fruits and vegetables and protection against cancer.Unlike case-control studies, cohort studies, which follow large groups of originally healthy individuals for a period of time, generally give more dependable information than case-control studies because they don't rely on information from history. And, in general, data from cohort studies haven't constantly shown that a diet rich in fruits and vegetables prevents cancer. For example, over a 14-month period in the nurses' health study and the health professionals' follow-up study, men and women with the highest input of fruits and vegetables(8 servings a day) were just as likely to have developed cancer as those who ate the smallest diurnal servings (under 1.5). A meta-analysis of cohort

studies found that advanced fruit and vegetable input didn't drop the risk of death from cancer. A more likely possibility is that some types of fruits and vegetables may protect against certain cancers.A study by and associates followed a nurses' health study ii cohort of 90,476 premenopausal women for 22 times and found that those who ate the most fruit during adolescence (about 3 servings a day) compared with those who ate the smallest inputs (0.5 servings a day) had a 25 percent lower risk of developing breast cancer. There was a significant reduction in breast cancer in women who had eaten advanced inputs of apples, bananas, and grapes,during nonage, and oranges during early adulthood. Farvid and associates followed 90,534 premenopausal women from the nurses' health study ii over 20 times and found that advanced fiber inputs during adolescence and early adulthood were associated with a reduced risk of breast cancer later in life. When comparing the highest and smallest fiber inputs from fruits and vegetables, women with the highest fruit fiber input had a 12 percent reduced risk of breast cancer; those with the highest vegetable fiber input had an 11 percent reduced risk. After following 182,145 women in nurses' health studies i and ii for 30 times, farvid's platoon also found that women who ate more than 5.5 servings of fruits and vegetables each day(yellow/ orange vegetables) had a 11 lower risk of breast cancer than those who ate 2.5 or smaller servings. Vegetable input was explosively associated with a 15-fold lower risk of estrogen receptor-negative tumors for every two fresh servings of vegetables eaten daily. An advanced input of fruits and vegetables was associated with a lower risk of other aggressive tumors, including hereditary and rudimentary tumors.
A report by the world cancer research fund and the american institute for cancer research suggests that non-starchy vegetables, such as lettuce and other leafy greens , broccoli, bok choy, cabbage, as well as garlic, onions, and the like, and fruits "presumably" cover against several types of cancers, including those of the mouth, throat, voice box, esophagus, and

stomach. Fruit presumably also protects against lung cancer. Specific factors in fruits and vegetables may also be protective against cancer. For example, a line of research stemming from a finding from the health professionals follow-up study suggests that tomatoes may help cover men against prostate cancer, especially aggressive forms of it. One of the colors that give tomatoes their red tinge lycopene   could be involved in this defensive effect. Although several studies other than the health professionals study have also demonstrated a link between tomatoes or lycopene and prostate cancer, others haven't or have set up only a weak connection. Taken as a whole, these studies suggest that increased consumption of tomato-based products(especially cooked tomato products) and other lycopene-containing foods may reduce the incidence of prostate cancer. Lycopene is one of several carotenoids(compounds that the body can turn into vitamin a) set up in brightly multicolored fruits and vegetables, and research suggests that foods containing carotenoids may protect against lung, mouth, and throat cancer. But more research is demanded to understand the exact relationship between fruits and vegetables, carotenoids, and cancer.

Diabetes - Some research looks specifically at whether individual fruits are associated with a risk of type 2 diabetes. While there isn't an abundance of research into this area yet, the primary results are compelling. A study of health professionals found that greater consumption of whole fruits, especially blueberries, grapes, and apples, was associated with a lower risk of type 2 diabetes. Another important finding was that higher consumption of fruit juice was associated with an advanced risk of type 2 diabetes. Also, a study of over 70,000 women aged 38–63 who were free of cardiovascular diseases , cancer, and diabetes showed that consumption of green, leafy vegetables and fruit was associated with a lower risk of diabetes. While not conclusive, research also indicated that consumption of fruit juice may be associated with an increased risk among women. A study of over 2,300 Finnish men showed that vegetables and fruits, especially berries, may reduce the risk of type 2 diabetes.

Weight - data from the nurses' health studies and the health professionals' follow-up study show that women and men who increased their inputs of fruits and vegetables over a 24-hour period were more likely to have lost weight than those who ate the same quantity or those who dropped their input. Berries, apples, pears, soy, and cauliflower were associated with weight loss, while starchy vegetables like potatoes,corn,and peas were linked with weight gain. Still, keep in mind that adding further produce to the diet won't inescapably help with weight loss unless it replaces another food, such as the refined carbohydrates of white bread and crackers.

Gastrointestinal health - Fruits and vegetables contain inedible fiber, which absorbs water and expands as it passes through the digestive system. This can calm the symptoms of a perverse bowel and, by driving regular bowel movements, relieve or help with constipation. The bulking and softening action of insoluble fiber also decreases pressure inside the intestinal tract and may help with diverticulosis. Eating fruits and vegetables can also keep your eyes healthy and may help with two common aging-related eye conditions cataracts and macular degeneration, which torment millions of Americans over the age of 65.

How to improve digestion through diet

To maintain good health, including a healthy digestive system, it's important to follow a balanced, healthy diet that includes a range of foods. It's also important to make life changes, such as avoiding smoking and staying active.

The Digestive System

The digestive system runs from the mouth to the anus and includes the stomach, the large and small intestine, and a number of apparent organs, including the salivary glands, liver, gallbladder, and pancreas. The purpose of the digestive system is to turn food and liquid into the structural blocks that the body needs to serve effectively. To do this, it produces and utilizes a variety of enzymes and other substances that aid digestion(breaking food down into lower moles). The amount of time food takes to digest goes thus: 2 hours through the stomach, 2 hours through the small intestine, and another 20 hours through the large intestine and rectum, making it a total of 24 hours to digest . The length of the digestive tube from mouth to anus is 9 measures on average. Each day, roughly seven liters of fluid are buried by the digestive system and its appurtenant organs. It's important to note that the words "intestine" and "bowel" are interchangeable. When the system works correctly, food is broken down so that nutrients can be absorbed and unwanted products excreted. When one or more of the functions of the digestive system fail, symptoms and diseases can develop. There are numerous different processes that contribute to a functioning and effective digestive system.

 Ingestion(putting food in your mouth)
Mechanical digestion(chewing and food being churned inside the digestive tract)
Chemical digestion(digestive enzymes and substances breaking down food) and Immersion (molecules passing from the digestive system into the body)
Making and passing droppings(feces)

Key Digestive System Components

 Mouth : The beginning of the digestive tract. food is put into the mouth and broken down by biting. This is called mechanical digestion. Colorful enzymes are buried to help with this breakdown, including saliva, or "saliva amylase', which is involved in the digestion of carbohydrates into lower chains and simple sugars. This is called chemical digestion.

Esophagus : Ingested food is swallowed and transported from the mouth to the stomach.

Stomach : Churning and mixing movements occur due to muscle condensation, continuing the process of mechanical digestion. Chemical digestion happens in the stomach. The food is mixed with gastric authorities and numerous digestive enzymes to help break down carbohydrates, proteins, and fats.

Hydrochloric acid is also released, which provides an acidic environment to help enzymes work and also kills some unwanted bacteria.

 Small intestine : The main function of the small intestine is to absorb nutrients and minerals. About 90 percent of digestion and immersion occur here, including the digestion of proteins, fats, and carbohydrates. Food is moved through the small intestine by coordinated condensation (called peristalsis) of the intestine wall, which occurs in a surge syndrome traveling down from one section to the next. The condensation occurs behind the ball of food (the bolus), forcing it through the digestive system.

Large intestine : The important function of the large intestine is to clear the water stored in it; this hardens the coprolite so it can be excreted from the body via the rectum and anus.

Accessory organs : The liver has numerous functions, which include helping with digestion, storing energy for the body(glycogen), helping the blood to clot, and removing or recycling alcohol, toxins and medications from the body. The liver also makes bile, which is stored in the gallbladder before passing into the small intestine, where it aids in fat digestion.

The pancreas has two main functions ; The product of digestive enzymes, which pass into the small intestine to help the chemical digestion of food, and the product of certain hormones, such as insulin, which help control blood sugar situations. The factors of the digestive system healthy eating

Why is healthy eating important?

Eating a healthy and varied diet can improve general well-being. Good nutrition is essential to gaining the nutrients demanded to keep the body healthy, as well as to avoid substances that may be dangerous. Having a healthy diet and doing regular exercise can help you achieve and maintain a healthy body weight. A healthy diet is also important to help reduce the risk of developing certain long-term conditions, such as diabetes, heart disease, and strokes. Also, it may reduce the risk of developing certain cancers and types of madness. Again, a poor diet can lead to weight gain and an increased risk of developing certain long-term conditions. Any of these health conditions can lead to a poor quality of life and other health complications, which can ultimately affect a dropped life expectation.

What's a healthy diet?

A healthy diet means a balanced diet. It involves eating a range of different foods from a variety of food groups in acceptable portion sizes. There are five different food groups: starchy foods(bread,rice, pasta, potatoes, and cereals); protein foods(meat, fish, eggs, and beans); dairy foods(milk, cheese, and yogurt); fruits and vegetables; and oils and spreads. One single food group cannot provide everything demanded for good health; Choosing a variety of foods from each group can help achieve a healthy, balanced diet. Starchy foods, vegetables, and fruit should make up the bulk of recipes. Fiber isn't just important for good gut health and functioning; it's also associated with a lower risk of cardiovascular diseases , type 2 diabetes, and bowel cancer. Starchy foods should be eaten regularly, and you should aim to include one portion with each meal. Where possible, advanced-fiber starchy foods, such as the whole grain versions of bread ,rice, other grains(barley, oats, buckwheat, bulgur,etc.), and breakfast cereals should be consumed. Beans, seeds, and nuts are also good sources of fiber and can help increase the amount, as well as the variety, of fiber we consume. The recommendation is to eat 30 grams of fiber a day, but most people only eat an average of 18 grams a day. It's advisable to increase the quantity of fiber consumed gradually and to drink plenty of fluids. There are different types of fiber, and each type behaves differently in your gut. Some types of fiber help make your coprolite bigger and easier to pass, which might help avoid constipation. Other types of fiber are digested(broken down) by your gut bacteria, producing substances that can be beneficial to your gut health. They might also produce gasses, which can cause bloating. People respond differently to different types of fiber, and it's worth noting that numerous foods contain more than one type of fiber. High-fiber foods are also dietary because they've got a lower glycemic index. The glycaemic index is a measure of the rate at which certain foods cause blood sugar to rise after they've been eaten. High-glycaemic-indicator foods such as sweets and white(refined) starchy foods release a lot of sugar quickly, which your body has to use up or, else, store as fat.

A certain quantity of protein is demanded and can be obtained from numerous different sources, including beans,fish, eggs, and meat. Protein should be eaten in moderation. To avoid redundant fat, choose lean meat or remove redundant fat and the skin from chicken. An example of calcium is dairy food. Calcium is required for healthy breasts and teeth, and it's recommended to have three servings a day from this food group. Only a small proportion of foods should be made up of fatty and sugary foods. to maintain a healthy diet and life, In addition to eating the correct foods, it's also important to be aware of other factors. These include maintaining a fluid input of around two liters per day.

Monitoring portion sizes : It can be easy to get into the habit of eating large portions. A rule of thumb for a meal is a fist-sized portion of carbohydrate and a palm-sized portion of protein. Minimizing sugary drinks, including fruit juice. Limiting alcohol input to 14 weekly units for men and women. Avoiding or reducing the input of certain foods, such as sweets, cakes, crisps, chocolate, and processed meat.
Aim for less than six grams of salt per day, And try to avoid adding salt to food.
Eating at least five portions of fruit and/or vegetables per day eat at least two portions of fish per week, one of which should be oily (e.g., mackerel, trout, sardines, kippers, or fresh tuna). replacing saturated fat with polyunsaturated or monounsaturated fat

Can a vegetarian diet be healthy?

A balanced vegetarian diet can be veritably healthy, particularly if acceptable quantities of food such as beans, lentils, cheese, and eggs are included to provide the necessary protein. But following a veritably restrictive diet can lead to nutrient scarcity, so if you choose to follow a strict diet that excludes all animal products, it may be wise to take vitamin supplements to avoid vitamin scarcity. It may also be worth consulting a dietitian.

Is a' clean diet' healthy?

There are numerous exemplifications of 'clean diets' on the internet and in the media. Still, as with all extreme diets, you have to be veritably careful that you don't reduce or remove essential food groups, as this can lead to malnutrition and health problems in the long term. For most people, following a well-balanced diet and lifestyle is more than enough to ensure good ongoing health.

Food Monitoring: How And Why?

Food monitoring can be a useful way to keep track of what and how important you're eating. It can be useful to keep a food journal and, at the end of the day, record what you have eaten, including snacks and drinks. It can help people identify areas of their diets that could be improved or changed to help them achieve a healthier diet, a healthier life, and weight loss or gain if demanded. Food and symptom monitoring can also be useful if you're suffering from digestion or gut issues to help identify possible detection foods.

Can stress affect my diet?

Stress is a normal response from your body to help you handle delicate levels or pitfalls. Temporary stress isn't generally a problem, but being constantly stressed can lead to stress-related symptoms and affect your health, including the health of your digestive system. Stress can also have an impact on your diet by making you miss meals or consume unhealthy foods. The gut and the brain are nearly linked and can affect one another. Persisting with a balanced, healthy diet during stressful times might help alleviate some of the symptoms of stress. It's worth exploring ways to manage stress, and there are a number of approaches and ways described online and in books. A starting point could be the nhs choices website, which has a section on meeting and managing stress.

Food Hygiene : How Important Is Food Hygiene?

Poor hygiene can clearly increase your chance of getting food poisoning. Food poisoning is generally a short-lived illness, but it can be veritably unwelcome while it lasts. Always wash your hands after visiting the restroom and before handling food. Care should be taken with the storage of food, particularly in hot weather. Certain foods, especially raw meat, must be kept covered, separated from other foods, and well cooled. It's best practice to follow the guidance handed by food manufacturers"use by and' best before 'dates. While some of these are used to specify when the food will be best, it can be risky to eat meat after the given date. When reheating food, make sure it's briskly all the way through (e.g., into the middle of a pie or down to the breast in a chicken leg) to kill all bacteria. However, don't eat it if it's a cold wave or you can see blood. This is particularly important when using a microwave oven or barbecue.

When Are You Supposed To See A Gp About Stomach Problems

All of us have short-lived gut problems from time to time. For the most part, this settles down by itself and should give no cause for concern. Still, you should see your gp about an unforeseen but patient change in the syndrome of how your intestines work, bleeding from the back passage, adding heartburn, indigestion, or stomach pain, losing weight suddenly ,unexpectant vomit and difficulty swallowing. All these are especially true if you have a family history of significant gut aches. You should also see your gp if you have been taking a remedy obtained from a drugstore for more than 2 weeks without any enhancement in your symptoms.

Exploring Diets : Finding What Works For You

Exploring different diets and deciding what works for you can be a fascinating trip. It's all about discovering what makes you feel best and finding a balance that suits your life. There are numerous resources available, like books, websites, and nutritionists, that can give guidance on different diets and help you navigate the options. Remember to hear your body and make choices that align with your particular preferences and health goals. It's all about chasing what works for you.

The Mediterranean diet is about eating lots of fruits, veggies, whole grains, and healthy fats like olive oil. You can enjoy fish, poultry, and dairy in moderation while limiting red meat and processed foods.

Ketogenic diet focuses on high-fat foods, moderate protein, and veritably low carbs. This type of diet strives to put your body in a state of ketosis, where it burns calories for energy. Sources: avocados, nuts, , and low-carb veggies.

The Paleo diet mimics what our ancestors ate during the stone age. It includes lean meats,fish, fruits, veggies, nuts, and seeds. You will avoid processed foods, grains, and dairy.

Vegan diet is all about plant-based foods and saying no to animal by products. Load up on fruits, veggies, whole grains, legumes, nuts, and seeds.

Creating A Personalized Diet Plan: The Best Diet That Works For You

The good news is that you do not need weeks' worth of expensive set frozen meats or a militant eating and exercise program to drop the weight. If you bristle at the idea of complying with someone else's idea of how you should exfoliate pounds, indeed, a slight drop in calories, rather on a plan that meets nutritive requirements, is all it takes. "One diet isn't inescapably any more successful than the next," says Joy

Bauer, MS, RD, author of "Your Inner Skinny". Four steps to Thin Forever "we know from research studies that nearly any plan that reduces calorie input results in weight loss, whether it's high-carbohydrate, low-carbohydrate, high-protein, or low-fat."

Weight loss will not last unless you change your eating and exercise habits for good in a way that matches with your food preferences, schedule, and life. dieter, let's get personal. Before you begin designing your own diet plan, some tone-reflection is in order. "Knowing who you're and what you need is the most important information you can have when it comes to losing weight, eating healthy, and changing your life," says Heather K. Jones, RD,co-author of What is your diet type? use the power of your personality to discover the best way to lose weight. "Our personalities explain why some approaches to weight control work while others fail." Jones says overeating takes more than restraint and that people who successfully lose weight and keep it off have simply discovered which approaches work for them and their unique personalities. 6 crucial questions to answer in order to design your own diet. Bauer and Jones advise asking yourself the following six questions: Do you prefer to eat three, five, or eight meals a day? Once you determine your eating schedule, divide your calories accordingly.

How much time will you devote to food medication? If you detest cooking or have limited time, you will need to simplify the medication of healthy, fresh, and lightly processed d foods. What type of support, and how much, do you need? Everyone needs some guidance to succeed, especially when the original enthusiasm for changing bad habits begins to wane. Family and musketeers, online weight loss communities, and diet communities can help you when you are tempted to ditch your healthier diet and exercise program.

Do you love to dine out? you will need to regard eatery food by seeking out the calorie counts of the foods you eat most frequently.

Will you bear a daily treat to feel satisfied? If you cannot live without something special every day, reserve 100 calories for a single-serve package of cookies or chips or for a frozen treat, like a fudge bar.

How much exercise can you do nicely? experts recommend at least 30 minutes a day of moderate physical exertion, such as walking, on most days of the week, but you may have to make up for that, especially if you are not physically active.

Calculating calories for weight loss

Diets do not work unless you run a calorie deficit by eating less energy than you burn. Most healthy people without habitual conditions can safely drop no more than two pounds a week on a balanced diet. Clinging to a daily calorie budget for weight loss is the crux of any successful do-it-yourself diet plan. Your calorie allowance is based on your age, sex, physical exertion level, and daily weight loss goals. Once you have calculated your calorie position, the next step is figuring out what to eat for weight loss. Bauer says the best diet plans are grounded in whole foods, such as vegetables, fruits, whole grains, lean protein, and low-fat dairy foods, because they lay the foundation for a continuance of healthy eating.

How to design your daily meal and snacks

You know how many servings from each of the food groups you need. Now you need to decide how to combine them to make healthy, satisfying treats and snacks that keep temptation at bay. Here are some introductory rules.

Have at least three meals a day. Eating on a regular basis prevents extreme hunger, which can annihilate your resolve to eat better and exercise more. stay fuller for longer by combining protein(set up in the highest quantities in foods from the milk and meat/sugar food groups) with fiber(set up in whole grains, vegetables, fruit, and legumes) at every meal and snack. Eating a calorie-free yogurt and an apple or a hard-boiled egg is more pleasant than spending the same number of calories on soda pop crackers, which are veritably low in fiber and devoid of protein.

Conserve calories. Choose the smallest-calorie choices from each food group. For example, opt for 1 reduced-fat milk or fat-free milk rather than full-fat; 93 lean ground beef rather than 85; and light popcorn rather than popcorn smothered in butter. Help portion distortion at home, and each food fits into a balanced weight control plan, but proper portions are paramount. Most people rarely go overboard on carrot sticks and celery, but it's a different story when it comes to cheese, pasta, fatty red poultry , and other favorite foods. Still, most of us are: invest in a dependable kitchen scale and measuring cups. If you are uncertain what constitutes reasonable serving sizes, let's face it. However, learn how to compare correct portion sizes to everyday objects, such as a baseball, if perfection is not your style. Right eyeballing portions is particularly helpful when dining out.

Creating your own diet plan is a great way to achieve weight-loss goals and understand the combination of nutrition and calories you need on a daily basis. In this composition, I'll explain How to calculate your needs, design a diet plan that supports your life and goals, and track your progress. Determine your calorie need with a calorie calculator and acclimate your diet, as demanded, to meet your preference. Produce a balanced diet to get the nutrition you need. Incorporate a healthy blend of protein, fruits, veggies, grains, dairy, and carbs into your diet. Track your progress by importing and measuring yourself daily. make dietary adaptations as you learn further about what works for your body.

- Calculating your nutritional requirements determines how many calories you need to eat daily. Your calorie need input depends on your age, sex, weight, height, and physical extension level. Generally, the more active you are, the more calories you will need to maintain your current weight. use this handy calorie calculator to quickly assess your calorie requirements. The US government recommends between 1,600 and 3,200 calories per day for adults. On average, most adults need about 2,000 calories. Generally speaking, the recommended calorie input is 2,000 calories a day for women and 2,500 for men. Exercise levels have a huge impact on the number of calories you can consume. For example, if you sit for the majority of the day, you might only be able to eat 1,800 calories without gaining weight. However, you might need 2,200 if you are veritably active.

- Set a reasonable weight-loss goal and a time frame to achieve it.

  As you are considering a long-term weight loss thing, keep in mind that losing more than 1–2 pounds a week is not healthy for you. Set yourself up for success by choosing a weight-loss thing that is both safe and attainable. For example, you might decide that your goal is to lose 15 pounds(7 kg) in 3 months. that the amount of weight and time frame are impeccably reasonable. You could indeed break that down into monthly goals. Strive to lose 7 lbs(3 kg) in the first month of dieting and 4 lbs(2 kg) for each of the reminders of the last 2 months. Set a daily sweet plan that will help you meet your weight-loss goal. Using your daily calorie needs as your base, figure out how many calories you need to cut to achieve your goal. That way, you can predicate your food choices around these specific figures and produce a diet that works for you. To lose 1 pound (0.45 kg) per week, cut 500–750 calories from your calorie diet. This is a great thing for weight loss. To lose 2 pounds (0.91 kg) per week, cut 1,000–1,500 calories per day. Trying to lose more than 2 pounds (0.91 kg) a week is drastic and potentially unhealthy. For instance, to lose 2 pounds (0.91 kg) in a week, you would have to cut 7,000 calories from your daily diet, which is relatively extreme.

- Focus on eating a balanced diet to get the nutrients you
  need.
  A good diet needs variety and balance and should
  include a healthy blend of protein, fruits, veggies,
  grains, dairy, and carbs.Aim to get 10–35 of your daily
  calories from protein. Eating protein-rich foods like
  beans, eggs, fish, legumes, poultry, milk, nuts, and soy
  helps you grow, tone, form, and develop. 2 cups(400 g)
  of fruit per day.Fruits contain vitamins and antioxidants;
  they can reduce the risk of health issues and are essential
  to a balanced diet. 2–3 cups (400–600 g) of veggies(
  fresh, frozen, or canned) a day. Vegetables contain loads
  of vitamins, potassium, fiber, and multitudinous health
  benefits. 5–8 ounces of complex carbs a day. You need
  carbohydrates for energy and to bolster your immune
  system. 3 cups(600 g) of any calcium-rich dairy per
  day. choose fat-free or low-fat milk, cheese, or lactose-
  free dairy.
- Increase your protein input to lose fat. Some studies
  showed that people who double their protein intake lose
  more weight via fat. To determine the quantity of
  protein you need, weigh yourself, multiply by 0.36, and
  also multiply that number by 2. The result is the quantity
  of protein you should get in grams to lose fat. For
  smaller calories, aim for proteins lower in fat. For
  example Milk: 149 calories for 8 grams of protein
   Eggs: 78 calories and 8 grams of protein per egg
  Greek yogurt: 100 calories and 15–20 grams of protein
   Cottage cheese: 100 calories for 14 grams of protein,
  and
  Edamame: 100 calories and 8 grams of protein.
- Incorporate low-calorie, complex carbs into your diet.
  Carbs are occasionally allowed to be " the adversary" by
  people trying to lose weight, but they play an important
  part in your health,especially in furnishing you with the
  energy to get through your day. Choose complex carbs

that are lower in calories to get the most value out of your foods. Complex carbs contain foods that are in their whole, unprocessed form. Foods in this order include fruits, vegetables, whole grain foods, oatmeal, and legumes. Simple carbs are sugars and starches that have been refined and stripped of their natural fiber and nutrients. Includes white bread, white rice, white pasta,etc. Lower-carb diets help with not only weight loss, but they've been shown to help lower blood pressure and blood sugar, as well as reduce the risk of heart disease.

- Reach for healthy fats over trans and saturated fats. Fats frequently get a bad name because of their association with actual body fat. There are still good fats that are absolutely essential to functions in your body, like maintaining body temperature and combating fatigue. Depending on the authority, fats should make up 30 percent or less of your diet. Knowing which fats can help a diet be successful, check the nutrition marker and ingredients list if you are eating packaged foods. Good fats come from a variety of sources, like sesame, olive, and canola canvases, soy beans, and nuts. You should also get omega-3 fatty acids from fish like salmon and tuna. Bad fats(trans and saturated) can cause cardiovascular diseases and diabetes. These fats are frequently in processed oil form or solid at room temperature, like red meat fat, shortening, and butter.

- Limit your input of salt and sugar.
Too much salt(sodium) leads to fluid retention, which causes stress on the heart and can lead to high blood pressure, heart complaint,or stroke. Also, excess sugar leads to obesity and a litany of health-related issues. Limit sodium to 2,300 mg or less per day. high-sodium foods to watch out for include pizza, soups, taco mixes, and salad dressing. Reduce sugar intake to 36 and 24 grams for males and females, respectively. Added sugars

go by a variety of names, with numerous sounding the same: dextrose, fructose, lactose, maltose, and sucrose. Other common sources are maple syrup, raw sugar, corn syrup, powdered sugar, brown sugar, and granulated sugar.

- Create healthy recipes and make a protein-rich breakfast to help you feel full longer. You will have more energy, lift up your metabolism, and feel full for longer. You can use this tool to help you find healthy breakfast fashions.

There are many great options to get you started. Add-in tablespoon) of oatmeal with delicious add-ins. Blend 1 cup(128 g) of oatmeal, 1 tbsp (15 ml) of peanut butter, and 1/4 mug(32 g) of raisins for a quick, easy meal,add 1 cup(240 ml) of orange juice for a healthy drink.

 Scramble 2 eggs with 2 tbsp low-fat milk, using 1 tsp (4.9 ml) vegetable oil. Add 2 turkey sausage, one slice of whole wheat toast, and 1 teaspoon (15 ml) of jelly. Drink 1 cup(240 ml) of recently squeezed orange juice.

Breakfast burrito. Put the sauteed tofu in an 8-inch flour tortilla with ¼ cup(32 g) of black beans and 2 tbsp (30 ml) of salsa. Wash it down with 1 cup (240 ml) of low-fat milk.

Eat a light lunch that includes veggies and lean proteins. There are numerous creative ways to make delicious lunches that energize you for the rest of the day. Try using this great resource to find healthy lunch recipes. There are many great examples : Green salad - put 3 ounces of tuna with 1 cup(128 g) of romaine lettuce, ¼ cup(32 g) of sliced carrots, and 2 tablespoons (30 ml) of vinaigrette dressing. Brace it with a slice of whole-wheat bread with 1 tsp(5 g) of margarine,drink 1 cup(240 ml) of low-fat milk.

Veggies peanut butter and banana sandwich - Combine 2 tablespoons of peanut butter and one medium banana on two slices of whole-wheat bread . Add ½ cup(64 g) of celery sticks for veggies and 1 cup (240 ml) of low-fat milk for the beverages.

Roast beef sandwich - Use 2 of lean roast beef between 2 slices of whole-wheat bread. Put in sliced tomato pieces, romaine lettuce, and 1 tbsp (15 ml) of mayo. Have ½ cup (32 g) of carrot sticks as a side. Add 1 cup(128 g) of sliced apple with a tablespoon of peanut butter for dessert.

Fix up a balanced diet with a blend of carbs, protein, and veggies. Produce some simple, family-friendly fashions sure to hit the health, diversity, and taste marks. Check out the options below and use this tool to find healthy regal fashions to try out. Red hot fusilli pasta - sauté 2 garlic cloves and ¼ cup(32 g) of parsley in 1 tbsp (15 ml) of olive oil. Add 4 mugs of diced tomatoes along with 1 tbsp(15 g) of basil, 1 tbsp(15 g) of oregano, 1/4 tsp (1.5 g) of salt, and ground red pepper. Cook the fusilli pasta(4 cups) and add 2 tablespoons (30 g) of shredded parmesan cheese to cook and cook ½ cup(64 g) of green peas as a side.

 5 ounces of chopped pork chops and a baked potato - Pan fry a 5-ounce pork chop and eat it alongside a baked potato with 2 tablespoons of salsa on top. Brace it with a cabbage slaw of 1/2 mug(64 f) of green cabbage mixed with 1 tbsp (15 ml) of vinaigrette dressing.

steak and mashed potatoes - cook 5 oz. of lean beef and serve it with 1 cup (128 g) of mashed potatoes and 1 cup (128 g) of mixed frozen vegetables.

- Control your portions by measuring food

 Check the portion size for each item in your meal, which is generally listed on the packaging. Try to limit yourself to the suggested portion size so you know exactly how many calories you are eating. A small steak or hamburger is generally 3–4 ounces. chicken breasts are about 3 ounces. A single egg equals 1 ounce. A cup (

32 g) of cooked beans, peas, or tofu is about 1 ounce. Go easy on the peanut butter! 1 teaspoon is equal to 1 ounce.

- Choose wisely when eating out. When eating out, use healthy eating options handed down by restaurants to make it easier. Numerous restaurants have entire sections devoted to meals under a certain number of calories. However, try a health food finder website to narrow down your list to the most healthy options if you can't make up your mind.

- Pre-pack your meals to help you stay on track. Not only can preparing your recipes beforehand help you diet by keeping you on track, but it can also make cravings easier to contain since there's food on hand. One extra benefit is a potentially huge cost savings. As you are creating and packing your recipes, take the time to list the nutritional aspects to stay motivated and informed. Tracking your progress weighs yourself daily to track weight loss. Weigh yourself before starting, and pick out a day to measure your weight each week at the exact time, putting on the same clothes from the first week.

Be consistent to see the gradual changes. Track it graphically or with an app to see your graded improvement. Take your measures every 6 weeks. muscle weighs more than fat, so the scale may not show the entire picture. For example , the scale may not show a significant change in your weight, but you look more neat in the glass because you've toned up your muscles and shed fat. Seeing those measures shrink over time can be really motivating! Just as with your weight, take the same measures periodically to gain an understanding of the changes in your composition. Revisit your goals every month and make changes as demanded. Change small things and try new ones!. Determine what's working for you and what isn't, and make small variations to reach your goals. Indeed, small changes can have a significant impact over time. Be careful not to restrict yourself too drastically. Some studies suggest that the more restrictive the diet, the more likely negative feelings, poor eating habits, and an advanced weight will be associated. Award yourself for making progress. Some experts recommend rewarding yourself for hard work by steering away from food and doing commodities differently that make you happy, like getting a massage, buying a book, or seeing a movie. Some diets may indeed include sweets or desserts.

Meal Fix For Busy Lifestyles

You aren't alone if you've made sweats to change your diet only to throw out rotten produce that you never got around to eating. This can be a frustrating experience, but there are strategies that can help you avoid food waste and produce various and scrumptious recipes. There are benefits to meal prepping during the week and ways to make it happen.

Benefits of meal prep

When it comes to a busy life, meal prepping can be a time-saver, a stress-reliever, and a way to save money. Planning out your daily reminders can help you concentrate on work or day-to-day tasks. Preparing recipes for the week gives you the capability to concentrate on what needs to be done without the stress of cooking a meal. Choose a day during the week that works best for you. Choose your favorite dishes to make, or ask yourself many questions about the type of dishes you want to fix ahead of time. What recipes do you enjoy at that point(i.e vegetables or fruit)? .What are your top three favorite vegetables? Are there any vegetables or fruits you don't currently eat but would like to try?One or two new items can help you gradually expand your produce input and learn new food preparation skills as well.

Save time by preparing meals : Taking an hour or two earlier in the week to plan your breakfasts, lunches, or feasts is actually saving you time as the week goes on. When you have your food fixed, you know what's available for you to eat, allowing you to make one less decision during the day. When you have a busy week, it saves you time to have your menu planned out.

Meal fix and reduce stress : When you have your food ready in the morning of the week, this allows you to free up your studies, concentrate on other tasks, and get tasks done. Coming home after a long day and trying to figure out what to cook can be stressful. Add in later days at the office or hitting traffic on the way home, and your mealtime dinner can turn into a quick grab-and-go meal through the drive-through.

Planning your recipes, Using your slow cooker, or having dinner ready to toast up in the roaster can reduce any stress you may feel. You have the capability to come home or finish your day with a healthy, home-cooked meal.

Meal fix and saving money: One of the benefits of preparing food ahead of time is that you only buy what you need at the grocery store, which cuts down on food waste. Frequently, we buy food to eat, but in our busy lives, we forget what we've got to eat, and the fresh food we buy goes to waste. Learning to make recipes that use the same ingredients for multiple recipes helps you cut down on food waste because you know exactly what's in your pantry or fridge and how it's going to be used. Think of versatile ingredients that you can use for numerous different recipes. For example, you can eat up a quinoa enchilada dish, black bean burgers, and a quinoa veggie chili, all of which include similar ingredients but give you three recipes for the week(and are freezer-friendly too!).

How to make meal prep happen

Let's start with menu planning fundamentals. Your shopping list should include the ingredients for your future meals and snacks, omitting what you have on hand. Select seasonal produce for cost savings, flavor, and added health benefits. Create your list while in your kitchen and survey your pantry, refrigerator, and freezer, in addition to your spice cabinet. Prioritize replenishing items that are running low or close their expiration date, and clear space on refrigerator and pantry shelves for the new items. Making a list has been shown to help consumers acquire over 80 of the items they intended to buy, and lists are effective "external memory storehouse bias" that reduces the stress of shopping. Making a list helps you avoid unintended purchases, stick to your budget, and ensure you have what you need for those planned meals or snacks. Studies show that when we calculate our memory for grocery shopping, we end up with only a bit of those items. It is a simple thing to get attracted by the good advertising and marketing of packaged foods.

Recipes ideas for meals (Breakfast, lunch, and dinner)

Plan your meals ahead of time, and take some time to plan out your breakfast, lunch, and dinner dishes. your future self will thank you!

Ideas for breakfast

Make a batch of steel-cut oatmeal and portion it out for the week ahead. Have fresh fruit ready to go in your fridge to add in for a quick, healthy breakfast ready to go. make a batch of carrot cake oatmeal or blueberry baked oatmeal. Both recipes can be made ahead of time, portioned out, and stored in your refrigerator or freezer for a quick reheat and delicious breakfast idea! Prepare a fruit salad ahead of time. Enjoy a piece of whole-grain toast topped with a nut butter of your choice. Prepare a crustless quiche ahead of time. Use this spinach and mushroom quiche to make ahead and keep in your fridge for over 5 days.

Ideas for lunch

Prepare salads ahead of time. use glass jars to place your salad mixture in. Add in different types of veggies, with your salad dressing on the side of the dish. Mix them up when you are ready to eat them.

Roasted vegetable sandwiches. Quickly toss any vegetables in a bowl and stir-fry for 3–5 minutes until tender the night ahead. Using a whole-grain pita or whole-grain tortilla, add hummus, roasted veggies, and feta cheese for a healthy sandwich to take with you on the go. put together sandwiches for the night before.

Choose lean sandwich meats such turkey, chicken , tuna, or salmon, and use whole-grain bread.Instead of mayonnaise, try yellow mustard. Keep it on the side for when you're ready to eat. top with veggies such as spinach, tomatoes, and cucumbers, and pack other raw veggies on the side or a piece of fresh fruit.

Dinner ideas

Make a sheet-pan meal

Using salmon or chicken and vegetables of your choice, place on a sheet-pan and toss with olive oil, salt, and pepper. Roast for 20–30 minutes.

Burrito bowls

Skilled- up lean ground beef or lemon sautéed peppers with a tablespoon of olive oil for 5 minutes . Using brown rice and a can of drained black beans place them together in four holders to have feasts ready to go.

Plant-based Diet Benefits

A plant-based diet means eating more whole foods and shopping for fruits, vegetables, whole grains, legumes, nuts, and seeds. One of the best things about eating a plant-based diet is that you can design it to fit your life. For some, a plant-based diet excludes all animal products(also known as a vegan diet). For others, it's just about choosing foods from plant sources rather than from animal sources. It's a nice way to make plants a main part of your diet without fully eliminating dairy, eggs, meat, and fish(you can just eat less of these). Regardless of which variation you want to follow, there are some benefits to eating further.

health benefits of eating a plant-based diet

Better nutrition : Plants are healthy, and most of us do not eat the recommended quantity of fruits and veggies, so making the maturity of your diet plant based will increase your produce consumption. fruits and vegetables are good sources of fiber,vitamins, and antioxidants.

Fiber is a nutrient that most of us do not get enough of, and it has tons of healthy benefits. It's good for your heart, your gut, and your blood sugar. A 2020 review in clinical nutrition found that consuming a vegetarian diet was associated with a reduced risk of negative health issues when compared to an omnivorous diet.

A healthier heart : Eating a vegetarian diet may lower your risk of cardiovascular diseases and may improve other risk factors for heart diseases by lowering your blood pressure and cholesterol and perfecting your blood sugar control. Eating plant-based foods can also help quell inflammation, which raises your risk of heart diseases by promoting plaque buildup on your arteries.

Lower diabetes risk : Eating a vegetarian diet can help treat type 2 diabetes, according to a 2021 study published in advances in nutrition. This is because plant-based diets improve insulin perceptivity, help with weight management, and reduce your risk of cardiovascular disease. Plant-based foods also have more fiber than animal foods, and increased fiber input has been associated with a dropped diabetes risk, according to a 2020 study published in the journal of diabetes investigation.

Diabetes-friendly vegan recipes

Decreased cancer risk : Research consistently shows that regularly eating a plenitude of fruits, veggies, legumes, and grains i.e plants is associated with a lower cancer risk. Plus, those disease-fighting phytochemicals in plants have also been shown to help and thwart cancer. And, do not forget, studies also show an association between eating red and processed meats and an increased cancer risk, especially colorectal cancer. So there is benefit not only from eating more plants but also from replacing some lower-healthy foods with plant-based foods.

Ok, so you are inspired now, right? Let's turn that into action. For starters, aim to make sure half of your lunch and dinner plates are always filled with vegetables, and vary the variety and color of the veggies you choose but there is more that you can do.Try to incorporate some of these small(ish) changes.

- Seek out healthy fats : Unsaturated fats ,monounsaturated and polyunsaturated are the kind that are good for your heart. Most of the good food sources

for these come from plants. Olives and olive oil ;
avocado and its oil painting; nuts and their butters and
oils. Substitute these sometimes (or always, if you
prefer) for butter, ghee, or lard, and you are
automatically leaning toward more plants. Aim to
include plant sources of omega-3 fatty acids too, such as
flaxseeds and chia seeds.

- Eat vegetables at breakfast : Start with breakfast if you
  want to increase your veggie input. Since it's not a meal
  you'd generally think about as veggie-filled, adding
  some then makes it easier to hit your daily quota. Try
  adding spinach to your eggs, blending cauliflower in
  your smoothie, or eating a breakfast salad.

- Have a vegetarian dinner once a week. Generally, we
  put animal protein at the center of the plate at
  dinnertime, So going vegetarian one day a week is one
  way to cut back. However, also shift your perception
  and see if you can make animal protein more of a
  condiment than an anchor to your meal one night a
  week. If going meat-free for a meal feels like a stretch, a
  month of vegetarian feasts in 30 minutes

- Try fruits for desserts and snacks : Numerous types of
  desserts are generally made with animal products;
  butter and eggs are common ingredients in
  cookies,cakes, and ice cream. Switching over to fruit can
  occasionally satisfy your sweet tooth with whole food
  and also give you a redundant serving of plants.

- Try one new-to-you plant food a week. This is a great
  way to increase the quantity of food you are eating while
  also adding variety to your diet, which means you will
  be getting a different balance of good-for-you vitamins
  and minerals.

The bottom line : When eating a plant-based food, you will
probably reap benefits from cutting down on meat(plant foods
have lower saturated fat and generally smaller calories), but it
goes beyond what you are limiting. What you are eating and

adding to your diet is significant too. Eating more plants means getting more of those good-for-you vitamins, minerals, phytochemicals, and fiber, many of which are nutrients we generally fall short on.

Low-carb And Ketogenic Diet Benefits

Low-carb diets have been controversial for decades. Some people assert that these diets raise cholesterol and cause heart disease due to their high fat content. Still, in the most scientific studies, low-carb diets prove their worth as healthy and beneficial.

Here are 10 proven health benefits of Low-carb and Ketogenic diets.

Low-carb diets reduce your appetite : Hunger tends to be the worst side effect of dieting. It's one of the main reasons why numerous people feel miserable and ultimately give up. Still, low-carb eating leads to an automatic reduction in appetite. Studies consistently show that when people cut carbs and eat more protein and fat, they end up eating far fewer calories. Studies indicate that cutting carbs can automatically reduce your appetite and calorie intake.

Low-carb diets lead to more weight loss at first : Reducing calorie input is one of the easiest ways to lose weight. Studies illustrate that people on low-carb diets lose more weight quickly than those on low-fat diets, even when the ultimate goal is restricting calories. This is because low-carb diets act to remove redundant water from your body, lowering insulin levels and leading to rapid weight loss in the first week or two. In studies comparing low-carb and low-fat diets, people who limit their carbs occasionally lose 2–3 times as much weight without being empty. One study in fat adults set up a low-carb diet that was particularly effective for over six months compared to a conventional weight-loss diet. When the study was completed,the difference in losing weight during dieting was not important. In a time-long study of 609 fat grown-ups on low-fat or low-carb diets, both groups lost analogous

quantities of weight. Nearly without exception, low-carb diets
lead to further short-term weight loss than low-fat diets. Still,
low-carb diets feel like they lose their advantage in the long
term.

A greater proportion of fat loss comes from your abdominal
cavity : Where fat is stored determines how it affects your
health and your risk of diseases. The two main types are
subcutaneous fat, which is under your skin, and visceral fat,
which accumulates in your abdominal cavity and is typical for
most overweight men. Visceral fat is mostly found around your
organs. Excess visceral fat is associated with inflammation and
insulin resistance and may drive the metabolic dysfunction, so
common in the west today. Low-carb diets are veritably
effective at reducing this dangerous abdominal fat. In fact, a
greater proportion of the fat people lose on low-carb diets
seems to come from the abdominal cavity. Over time, this
should lead to a drastically reduced risk of heart disease and
type 2 diabetes. A large percentage of the fat lost on low-carb
diets tends to be dangerous abdominal fat that's known to cause
serious metabolic problems.

Triglycerides tend to drop dramatically : Triglycerides are fat
molecules that circulate in your bloodstream. It's well known
that high fasting triglyceride levels in the blood after a late fast
are a strong heart complaint risk factor. One of the main causes
of elevated triglycerides in sedentary people is carbohydrate
consumption, especially simple sugar fructose. When people
cut carbs, they tend to witness a veritably dramatic reduction in
blood triglycerides. On the other hand, low-fat diets frequently
cause triglycerides to increase. Low-carb diets are veritably
effective at lowering blood triglycerides, which are fat
molecules that increase your risk of heart disease.

Increased levels of good'S HDL cholesterol : high-viscosity
lipoprotein(HDL) is frequently called "good " cholesterol. The
higher your levels of HDL relative to "bad" LDL, the lower
your risk of heart complaint. One of the best ways to increase
"good" HDL levels is to eat fat, and low-carb diets include a lot

of fat. Thus, it's unsurprising that HDL levels increase
dramatically on healthy, low-carb diets, while they tend to
increase only relatively or indeed decline on low-fat diets.
Low-carb diets tend to be high in fat, which leads to an
impressive increase in "good " HDL cholesterol.

Reduced blood sugar and insulin levels : Low-carb and
ketogenic diets can also be particularly helpful for people with
diabetes and insulin resistance, which affect millions of people
worldwide. Studies prove that cutting carbs lowers both blood
sugar and insulin levels drastically. Some people with diabetes
who begin a low-carb diet may need to reduce their insulin
intake by 50 percent, almost immediately. In one study of
people with type 2 diabetes, 95 had reduced or eliminated their
glucose-lowering medications within six months. Still, talk to
your doctor before making changes to your carbohydrate input,
as your dosage may need to be adjusted to help hypoglycemic
if you take blood sugar medication.

May lower blood pressure : Elevated blood pressure, or
hypertension, is a significant risk factor for numerous
conditions, including heart disease, stroke, and heart failure.
Low-carb diets are an effective way to lower blood pressure,
which should reduce your risk of these conditions and help you
live longer. Cutting carbs leads to a significant reduction in
blood pressure, which should reduce your risk of numerous
common conditions.

Effective against the metabolic syndrome : Metabolic
syndrome is a condition largely associated with your risk of
diabetes and heart diseases . In fact, a metabolic syndrome is a
collection of symptoms, which include - abdominal obesity,
elevated blood pressure, high triglycerides and low "good"
HDL cholesterol levels. Still, a low-carb diet works
miraculously in treating all of these symptoms. Healthy low-
carb diets effectively reverse all five crucial symptoms of
metabolic syndrome.

Improved bad LDL"cholesterol levels : People who have high
"bad" LDL are much more likely to have heart attacks; still, the

size of the particles is important. lower particles are linked to a higher risk of heart diseases, while larger particles are linked to a lower risk. It turns out that low-carb diets increase the size of "bad" LDL particles while reducing the number of total LDL particles in your bloodstream. Similarly, lowering your carbohydrate input can boost your heart health. When you eat a low-carb diet, the size of your "bad" LDL particles increases, which reduces their harmful effects. cutting carbs may also reduce the number of total ldl particles in your bloodstream. Therapeutic for several brain disorders : Your brain needs glucose, as some of it can only burn this type of sugar. That's why your liver produces glucose from protein if you don't eat any carbs. Yet, a large part of your brain can also burn ketones, which are formed during starvation or when carbohydrate input is very low. This is the mechanism behind the ketogenic diet, which has been used for decades to treat epilepsy in children who don't respond to medicine. In one study, over half of the children on a ketogenic diet experienced a greater of less than 50 seizures, while 16 went seizure-free. Veritably low-carb and ketogenic diets are now being studied for other brain conditions as well, including Alzheimer's and Parkinson's. Low-carb and keto diets have proven to be beneficial in treating epilepsy in children and are being studied for their effects on other brain conditions.

Mindful Eating

Mindful eating starts with assessing your hunger, it also starts with taking a moment to listen to your body. Can mindfulness help you stop binge eating? you're not alone. Estimates suggest that people struggling to lose weight who are seeking help generally(between 25 and 30) suffer from cavity or other psychological disorders, leading to emotional and binge eating. That's no surprise, as evidence links restrictive diets, generally used in attempts to lose weight, as significant contributors to binge eating. Findings show it's possible to reduce the number of binge-eating occurrences and improve expressive feelings with the use of mindful eating strategies. Looking at your food is part of mindful eating. find a comfortable place to sit and enjoy taking in the sights and smells of the food you're eating. Looking at your food and smelling it actually stimulates the digestive system, getting your body ready to process the incoming food. You've presumably noticed this very process the last time you looked at delicious food and your mouth doused. That's saliva being made for preparation for you to eat.

Exclude distractions while you eat to help with weight loss. Avoiding distractions is the best way to be more aware of how you're eating. Studies have set up a wide variety of factors that can distract you from eating mindfully: computer games, listening to a story, background music, or other electronic devices. In fact, eating in competition with other tasks has been shown to increase food input about 15 more calories and an advanced consumption of fat.

Do pre-eaters gain further weight?

Being a fast eater may be a reason you or someone you love is struggling to manage your body weight. findings from a research study propose that people who eat faster are at higher risk for weight gain and obesity. Published in the journal clinical obesity, the study suggests eating faster puts you at a higher risk of obesity due to the delay in consumption of wholeness compared to when you eat slowly . The reason is explained by healthy living expert and registered dietician Kimberly Gomer, director of nutrition at the pritikin longevity center and spa. "Slow down; it takes 15 to 20 minutes for the stomach to tell the brain that you're full."

Can weight loss be done mindfully?

Digging your chopstick into that delicious food, you stuff it into your mouth, snappily bite it into bits, and as you're swallowing, you formerly have the coming forkful, staying impatiently by your lips. However, you may be eating too quickly, if that sounds like you. That nibble you just swallowed has a long way to go down your throat down the length of your esophagus and into your stomach. It takes a while. In your stomach, you have stretch receptors that smell food and send a message to your brain to tell you, "Thanks, I'm ok now; you can stop eating." it's possible to not pay attention to your stomach signals if you're eating during the course of getting distracted by phones, news, computer work, or driving. The average person takes 15 to 20 minutes to get a signal from their stomach. How long have you taken to eat ? Worse, how frequently have you quickly returned to get second helpings before staying long enough to allow your stomach to shoot you a message about how full you really are?

 How to eat slowly: "slow down; it takes 15 to 20 minutes for the stomach to tell the brain that you're full," notes Kimberly Gomer,R.D. "it's all about how you should eat and just what you should eat," explains kimberly Gomer,,R.D.

Nourishing Nutrition For Optimal Health :

Revitalizing Your Body

Superfoods And Functional Foods : Unleashing The

Nutritional Powerhouses

Here is a brief rundown on superfoods and functional foods. Superfoods are nutrient-dense foods that offer a range of health benefits. Examples include berries, leafy greens, nuts, and seeds. They are rich in antioxidants, vitamins and minerals which can help support your overall health. Functional foods, on the other hand, go beyond introductory nutrition. They contain bioactive composites that can have specific health benefits. For example, turmeric has anti-inflammatory properties, and probiotic-rich yogurt can promote gut health. Incorporating superfoods and functional foods into your diet can be a delicious way to boost your nutrition and support your well-being!.

Superfoods are types of foods that are packed with the highest density of nutrients and are the most beneficial for your body. While most non-processed foods benefit the body in some way, options that are considered superfoods are generally the healthiest foods available and are rich in more than one type of nutrient. Still, it's important to note that superfoods are only part of a balanced diet, not the only things you should be eating. A healthy diet should contain the correct portions of a variety of foods, not just large quantities of many of the" healthiest" options. They're especially high in nutrients that are hard to find in other foods, such as fiber, protein, antioxidants, and a variety of vitamins and minerals. Filling your diet with these types of foods can help give you further energy, help you maintain a healthy weight, and lower your risk for heart problems, cancer, obesity, and other health concerns that are generally associated with poor nutrition.

How does including superfoods in your diet benefit your body?

Although the name 'superfoods' makes them feel like commodities greater, eating a superfood-heavy diet basically just means making healthy choices. Eating more superfoods and elevating your diet can be achieved by knowing what foods to buy at the supermarket and adding those foods to your diet. Although you should not solely eat foods that are labeled as superfoods, there are numerous delicious and simple ways to add more of them to your balanced diet. Blending berries, spinach, other greens, and other supplements into smoothies is a delicious way to consume a variety of superfoods. Drinking green tea throughout the day also provides numerous benefits. Adding fruits and nuts to salads can increase their nutritive value, and applesauce can be used as a healthier substitute for sugar in a variety of baked goods.

Tip number one: Start small. Don't try to be a superhero yourself by incorporating all the superfoods at once. Start with one or two that you love, like blueberries or spinach, and work your way over from there.

Tip number two:Mix and match! Superfoods are like the spice rack of healthy eating, so don't be afraid to experiment with different combinations. Add chia seeds to your morning smoothie or top your salad with salmon for a delicious and nutritious meal.

Tip number three: Snack like a superhero! Numerous superfoods make great snacks on their own, like almonds or blueberries. Keep a store of them at your office or in your bag for a quick and healthy pick-me-up.

Tip number four: Try different recipes. Superfoods can be incorporated into a variety of fashions, from smoothies to salads to main dishes. Experiment with different fashions to find what works best for you.

 Tip number five Look for opportunities to add them to your meal. Look for opportunities to add superfoods to your meals whenever possible. For illustration, try adding spinach to your omelet or avocado to your sandwich.

Now, let's talk about some of the superfoods and their benefits. Blueberries are like little bombs of antioxidants that can improve cognitive function and reduce inflammation.

Spinach is a nutrient powerhouse that can ameliorate bone health and reduce inflammation. Salmon is a great source of omega-3 fatty acids, which can improve heart health and reduce inflammation. And chia seeds are fiber-rich little gems that can improve digestion and provide a good source of omega-3s and antioxidants.

 Lastly, let's dive into turmeric and its benefits.

 The bright, unheroic spice contains curcumin, which has important anti-inflammatory properties and may help enhance brain function and reduce the threat of habitual conditions. Add it to your curries, soups, and smoothies for an extra boost of superhero power.

Incorporating superfoods into your diet doesn't have to be a chore. With a little bit of creativity, a little bit of planning, and a whole cargo of fun, you can transfigure your recipes into succulent and nutritional superfood feasts.

Functional foods and their health benefits

Functional foods are ingredients that offer health benefits that extend beyond their nutritive value. Some types contain supplements or other fresh ingredients designed to enhance health. The concept began in Japan in the 1980s, when government agencies started approving foods with proven benefits in an effort to improve the health of the general population. Some examples include foods fortified with vitamins, minerals, probiotics, or fiber. Nutrient-rich ingredients like fruits, vegetables, nuts, seeds, and grains are frequently considered functional foods as well. Oats, for example, contain a type of fiber called beta-glucan, which has been shown to reduce inflammation, enhance vulnerable function, and improve heart health. Also, fruits and vegetables are packed with antioxidants, which are beneficial compounds that help protect against diseases.. Functional foods are foods that offer health benefits beyond their nutritive value. In addition to nutrient-rich ingredients like fruits and veggies, the order also includes foods fortified with vitamins, minerals, probiotics, and fiber.

Examples

Functional foods are generally separated into two orders: conventional and modified.

Conventional foods are natural, whole-food ingredients that are rich in important nutrients like vitamins, minerals, antioxidants, and heart-healthy fats. Meanwhile, modified foods have been fortified with fresh ingredients, such as vitamins, minerals, probiotics, or fiber, to increase a food's health benefits.

Here are some examples of conventional functional foods.
Fruits: berries, kiwi, pears, peaches, apples, oranges, and
bananas.
Vegetables: broccoli, cauliflower, kale, spinach, and zucchini.
Nuts: almonds, cashews, pistachios, macadamia nuts, and
Brazil nuts.
Seeds: chia seeds, flax seeds, hemp seeds, and pumpkin seeds.
Legumes: black beans, chickpeas, navy beans, lentils.
Whole grains: oats, barley, buckwheat, brown rice, and
couscous.
 Seafood: salmon, sardines, anchovies, mackerel, and cod.
Fermented foods: tempeh, kombucha, kimchi, kefir, and
sauerkraut.
Herbs and spices: turmeric, cinnamon, ginger, cayenne pepper.
Beverages: coffee, green tea, black tea
Then are some examples of modified functional foods.
Fortified juices, fortified dairy products (similar to milk and
yogurt), fortified milk alternatives (similar to almond, rice,
coconut, and cashew milk),
fortified grains (similar to bread and pasta), fortified cereal
and granola,fortified eggs.
Nutrient-rich foods like fruits, veggies, and legumes are
frequently considered functional foods, along with fortified
foods like juice, eggs, and cereal.
**Functional foods are associated with several potential
health benefits.**

- Prevention of nutrient scarcity : Functional foods are
  generally high in important nutrients, including
  vitamins, minerals, healthy fats, and fiber. Filling your
  diet with a variety of functional foods, including both
  conventional and fortified foods, can help ensure you get
  the nutrients you need and cover against nutrient
  scarcity. In fact, since the introduction of fortified foods,
  the frequency of nutrient scarcity has significantly
  dropped around the globe. For example, after iron-
  fortified wheat flour was introduced in Jordan, rates of

iron-insufficiency anemia among children were nearly cut in half. Fortification has also been used to help with other conditions caused by nutrient scarcity, including rickets, goiter, and birth defects.

- Protection against diseases : Functional foods provide important nutrients that can help protect against diseases. Numerous foods are especially rich in antioxidants. These molecules help neutralize dangerous compounds known as free radicals, helping to prevent cell damage and certain habitual conditions, including heart disease, cancer, and diabetes. Some functional foods are also high in omega-3 fatty acids, a healthy type of fat shown to reduce inflammation, boost brain function, and promote heart health. Other types are rich in fiber, which can promote better blood sugar control and protect against conditions like diabetes, obesity, heart disease, and stroke. Fiber may also help with digestive diseases, including diverticulitis, stomach ulcers, hemorrhoids, and acid reflux.

- Promote proper growth and development : Certain nutrients are essential to proper growth and development in babies and children. Enjoying a wide range of nutrient-rich functional foods as part of a healthy diet can help ensure that nutritive requirements are met. In addition, it can be beneficial to include foods that are fortified with specific nutrients that are important for growth and development. For instance, cereals, grains, and flours are frequently fortified with B vitamins like folic acid, which is essential for fetal health. Low levels of folic acid can increase the risk of neural tube defects, which can affect the brain, spinal cord, or spine. It's estimated that adding the consumption of folic acid could drop the frequency of neural tube defects by 50–70%. Other nutrients generally set up in functional foods also play crucial roles in growth and development, including omega-3 fatty acids, iron, zinc, calcium, and vitamin B12.

Uses

A balanced and healthy diet should contain different types of functional foods, including nutrient-rich whole foods like fruits, vegetables, whole grains, and legumes. Functional foods help with overall well-being and also provide the body with vitamins and minerals. Modified, fortified functional foods can also fit into a balanced diet. In fact, they can help fill any gaps in your diet to help with nutrient scarcity, as well as enhance your health by boosting your intake of important nutrients like vitamins, minerals, fiber, heart-healthy fats, or probiotics.

Functional foods can be used to boost your intake of important nutrients, fill any gaps in your diet, and support overall health. Functional foods are an order of foods associated with several important health benefits.

What's a fortified cereal?

Fortified foods are filled with vitamins and minerals that aren't present in them naturally. Fortification is meant to help problems with particular nutrients in common foods that adults and children generally eat, such as grains, milk, and juice. Cereal is one of the best-known types of fortified foods. For example, 1 cup(40 grams) of fortified total cereal boasts 40 mg of iron—100 of the daily value. As the same size serving of an unfortified wheat cereal meets only 10% of the DV, much of breakfast cereals' iron content may be due to fortification. It's important to cover your nutrient input, as numerous people in the United States don't consume enough iron, calcium, or vitamins A, C, D, and E.scarcity may lead to negative health effects. Breakfast cereals are generally fortified with the following nutrients: vitamin A thiamine (vitamin B1) riboflavin(vitamin B2) Niacin (vitamin B3) vitamin B6; vitamin B12; vitamin D folic acid zinc, iron and, calcium. Fortified cereals contain added vitamins and minerals to help absorb nutrients. Food manufacturers frequently fortify ready-to-eat,pre-packaged cereals, and occasionally hot cereals like oatmeal. Still, fortified cereals aren't inherently healthy. While some are made with whole grains and are high in fiber and protein, others contain almost no nutrients. You can distinguish the difference between a fortified cereal and a non-fortified one by checking the nutrients that would be added to the packaging. Frequently, below the component list, there's a list of vitamins and minerals used to fortify the product. Keep in mind that fortification varies by region. Fortified cereals are generally known to be found in western countries. What's more, certain countries, including the United States, Canada, Costa Rica, Chile, and South Africa, mandate the fortification of wheat flour with folic acid, so it's more common to find folic acid-enriched cereals in these places. Notably, cereals that are less heavily processed are less likely to be fortified. Num

Health benefits of fortified cereal

- Eating fortified cereal may help with nutrient scarcity : With advanced nutrient input, numerous people in the United States don't meet the nutritional recommendations for certain vitamins and minerals.As such, eating fortified foods may help. A recent study noted that eating fortified foods boosted the intake of folate and vitamins A and C. Some people, such as young children, vegetarian, and pregnant or breastfeeding women, may profit particularly from fortified cereals due to their increased nutrient requirements. That said, fortified foods may increase your threat of exceeding certain nutrient recommendations.

- Lower threat of birth defects : Fortifying cereal grains with folic acid, the synthetic form of folate, has successfully reduced the prevalence of neural tube defects, which are one of the most common birth defects in North America. Folate is a vitamin B important for proper growth and overall well-being. In fact, all women of working age are advised to consume 400 mcg of folic acid daily from fortified foods and/or supplements, as

well as eat folate-rich foods. Thus, fortified cereal may profit women who are or may become pregnant.
 Specifically, fortifying foods with folic acid has helped reduce the risks of birth defects.Potential downsides of fortified cereal ; While fortification can enhance nutrient content, cereal is still a processed food and isn't necessarily healthy.

- May be loaded with sugar and refined carbs : Numerous fortified cereals are high in added sugar and refined carbs, plus most people eat more than the recommended serving size. In fact, a study of 72 adults determined that people ate 200 of the labeled serving sizes on average. According to the American Heart Association(AHA), women and men should limit their daily input of added sugar to 25 and 37.5 grams, independently. This means that a bowl or two of fortified cereal could easily put you close to or indeed above your daily sugar limit. Not only do Americans tend to formally exceed guidelines for sugar input, but diets high in added sugars are also associated with an increased threat of habitual conditions like obesity, heart disease, and diabetes.

Misleading health claims
 Numerous manufacturers label their cereals with misleading health claims, similar to "low-fat" or"whole-grain." This is deceptive because the primary ingredients are generally refined grains and sugar. Research suggests that diets high in added sugar raise your risk of heart disease. Such misleading claims may lead people to consume foods that aren't healthy. What's more, numerous fortified cereals are marketed to children. Studies reveal that advertisements affect children's taste preferences and may contribute to the obesity threat. As such,you should read labels precisely to avoid any misleading claims. Fortified cereals are generally not as healthy as their packaging asserts, as numerous are high in added sugar and refined carbs. It's best to choose

cereals that are low in sugar and high in fiber. Look for types with less than 6 grams of sugar and at least 3 grams of fiber per serving. Fiber can help boost wholeness and reduce cholesterol, among other benefits. Since numerous cereals require protein, include a protein source to produce a more satisfying, balanced meal. Consider adding Greek yogurt, nuts, or peanut butter. Still, the best option for a nutrient-rich breakfast is whole, unprocessed foods, such as oatmeal, yogurt, fruit, or eggs. . Fortified cereals are generally eaten for breakfast and may help with certain nutrient shortages.

Gut-brain Connection : How Nutrition Impacts Mental Health And Energy

Nutrition plays a crucial role in the gut-brain connection and impacts both internal health and energy levels. A healthy diet with nutrient-rich foods can support a balanced gut microbiome, which can positively impact internal well-being. Certain nutrients, like omega-3 adipose acids, B vitamins, and antioxidants, have been linked to better mood and cognitive function. Also, stable blood sugar levels from a balanced diet can help sustain energy throughout the day.

Gut-brain Connection To Mental Health

Stomach problems are one of the most common symptoms of stress and anxiety. Experimenters have linked a connection between the gut and the brain. Like the brain, your gut is full of nerves called the enteric nervous system, or ENS, also referred to as the "alternate brain ". The enteric nervous system has the exact type of neurotransmitters and neurons fixed in your central nervous system. This connection between the brain and gut has effects on digestion, mood, and the way you think. ENS lines your entire digestive system with more than 100 million nerve cells forming two layers. It runs through the esophagus to the rectum.

How Your Gut and Brain Relate

Your alternate brain monitors and controls your digestion, from swallowing to the release of enzymes. It ensures the breakdown of food into small particles, controlling blood flow for nutrient absorption and elimination. For decades, experimenters thought that depression and anxiety contributed to people experiencing Irritable Bowel Syndrome (IBS) and functional bowel problems such as constipation, diarrhea, bloating, pain, and stomach upset. Still, some other research shows that ENS can be the cause. The ENS relates to the brain by going through the nervous system and your hormones. An exchange of information also takes place between your gut and the immune system, affecting your overall internal health. It's also believed to contribute to conditions like Parkinson's and Alzheimer's, autism, amyotrophic lateral sclerosis, multiple sclerosis, pain, and anxiety.

Stress-related gut symptoms and conditions

When you're nervous or anxious, your body releases some hormones and chemicals that enter the digestive system. This can have a big effect on the microorganisms that stay in your gut, helping in the digestion process while removing antibody products. A chemical imbalance can cause several gastrointestinal conditions, similar to indigestion. Stomach upset and diarrhea, irritable bowel syndrome (IBS),constipation, loss of appetite or unusual hunger and nausea .

How to improve Your Gut

If you want to improve your gut health, there are several things you can do.

- Effectively digest your food : After a meal, it's important to be in a relaxed state to produce the gastric juices needed to absorb food. Gastric juice is essential for the immersion of vitamins, minerals, and nutrients necessary to support a healthy body and brain.

- Mind what and how you eat : Eat healthy snacks and treats, and stay away from junk food. One way to do this is to prepare pre-planned meals, have some fruits, or have a granola bar to snack on when hungry. Also, take time when you eat to completely savor the food, enjoying every bite.
- Exercise : It can be hard to exercise regularly, but scheduling some exercise time can encourage you to work out. Alternatively, take a walk around your neighborhood. This can help you reduce stress and improve your physical and emotional well-being.
- Drink plenty of water : Aim to drink between six and eight glasses of water a day to boost the digestive process.
- Seek help. A therapist who specializes in anxiety can help you manage your chronic worry.

Food For Your Mental Health

The key to perfecting your gut health is knowing the types of foods that boost your gut health and internal health. Some of these foods include:

Fiber - Eating fiber improves memory and overall mood. It also reduces inflammation and oxidative stress by encouraging the microbiota. Foods rich in fiber include beans and legumes, oats, nuts, dark chocolate, fruits, and vegetables.

VitaminD - Vitamin D stabilizes your microbiome and decreases gastrointestinal inflammation. Some foods that have vitamin D include egg yolk, tuna, salmon, orange juice, and fortified milk. Protein - Proteins contain nitrogen, which reduces the amount of bad bacteria found in a microbiome. Eating protein may lower your feelings of depression because of the product of serotonin, which improves your mood. Good sources of proteins include eggs, milk, yogurt, lean beef, lemon, chicken, fish, broccoli, oats, and nuts.

Omega- 3s - Omega-3 fatty acids help reduce cholesterol levels, increase memory and cognitive function, and lower sugar levels.Sources of Omega 3 are walnuts, flax seeds, salmon, sardines, and mackerel.

Nutrients For Internal Clarity And Concentration

Your brain is hungry for nutrition. Indeed, though this organ makes up only 2% of your body's weight, it gobbles up 20% of its calories. However,if you like to stay sharper,more focused ,these five nutrients would help .

Lutein

This plant pigment is set up in every part of the brain, and it aids in literacy and memory. It's so important that a joint Abbott and University of Illinois Center for Nutrition, Learning, and Memory study set up that seniors with the highest blood lutein levels showed superior"crystalline intelligence," a measure of the capability to use skills and information acquired throughout the lifetime. In addition, exploration has shown that the amount of lutein in your eye positively relates to the processing speed in your brain. The top sources of lutein are spinach, kale, corn, pumpkin, sweet potatoes, avocados, and egg yolk.

DHA Omega- 3

Did you know that fat makes up nearly 60% of your brain? A good thing is to choose the healthiest fats possible, like docosahexaenoic acid(DHA). This omega-3 fat comprises 25 percent of the brain's fat, helping to reduce inflammation and foster communication between brain cells. Top sources for DHA fatty fish like salmon, tuna, and sardines The body can also make DHA from flaxseeds, walnuts, and soybeans.

B Vitamins

This family of vitamins protects the brain in multiple ways. B vitamins like thiamin and niacin help the brain metabolize nutrients for energy. Others, like vitamins B12 and folate, can help protect against dementia by breaking down homocysteine, a dangerous substance that may lead to Alzheimer's disease. The top sources of B vitamins are a balanced diet of lean meat,

poultry, fish, dairy, whole grains, fruits, and vegetables. However, consider a B12 supplement, as this vitamin is only found in animal foods, if you are a strict vegetarian or vegan.
Vitamin D

Helps keep your bones and heart strong. It may also help you maintain a sunnier disposition by helping brain cells produce mood-regulating neurotransmitters such as dopamine and serotonin. Top sources for vitamin D are trout, salmon, organ meats like liver, milk, fortified cereals, and eggs.

Protein Healthy muscles do not just keep you strong. They are also linked to better cognitive capacities in older people. Protein provides structure blocks that save muscle mass, which is especially important since most people begin to lose muscle as early as age 40. For optimum muscle health, aim for 25 to 30 grams of protein at every meal. Top sources for protein: lean meat, poultry, seafood, eggs, milk, yogurt, cheese, tofu, beans, and lentils.

The brain accounts for about 2 percent of your total body weight, but it uses 20 percent of your energy input, so it's essential to feed it the right foods every day. Expert nutritionists explain the best foods and vitamins for your brain. Glucose is your brain's preferred source of energy. Your brain uses up more energy during challenging mental tasks, so keeping blood glucose levels in an optimal position will help your cognitive function. Eating regular meals also helps. A balanced diet with carbohydrate foods including whole grains, vegetables, fruits, and legumes will give your brain a steady force of glucose and benefit your concentration. Dietary fat is important for brain function. and, in particular, the omega-3 fatty acids. Around 60 percent of the brain is made up of fat, and around half of that is omega-3 fatty acids. The long-chain omega-3 fatty acids set up in oily fish, such as salmon, trout, mackerel, and sardines, are viewed as particularly beneficial for maintaining normal brain function. Still, your body can convert the short-chain omega-3 fatty acids from some plant foods(although not veritably efficiently) into the long-chain omega-3 fatty acids if your diet doesn't include fish. These plant foods include walnuts, flax, hemp, chia, pumpkin seeds, and rapeseed oil.

The Best Foods For Your Brain

The brain requires a wide range of nutrients to function well. The best way to ensure you get all the essential nutrients is by eating a healthy and varied diet. A Mediterranean-style diet is thought to be particularly beneficial for brain health,good foods to include are:

All vegetables(especially green leafy vegetables such as kale, spinach, salads, and cooked greens),berries(including blueberries, blackberries, strawberries, and raspberries),a variety of different nuts and seeds,whole grains(such as oats, brown rice, quinoa), whole-wheat bread

and pasta, a variety of different legumes(beans, peas, and lentils), some lean meat, fish, if you're not vegan or plant-based.

Vitamin C :Vitamin C helps reduce tiredness and fatigue, so snacking on a piece of fruit, a berry smoothie, or a red pepper and tomato soup should help you feel more awake.

Vitamins B: Vitamin B help convert the food you eat into energy, so they're vital for getting energy to your brain. Vitamins B1, B2, B6, Folate, and Vitamin B12, for example, all play a crucial role in brain function. Pantothenic acid(or Vitamin B5) helps internal performance. Meat, eggs, wholegrain foods, and nearly all vegetables, in particular mushrooms and avocados, contain vitamin B5.

Calcium: Calcium contributes to the normal neurotransmission function of your brain, which helps pass messages between cells and is also allowed to be involved in your literacy and memory functions. Dairy products are a best source of calcium, but if you don't consume dairy, include non-dairy milk or yogurt with added calcium, tofu made with calcium sulfate or beans,chickpeas, sesame seeds, kale, spinach, and broccoli, which are also good sources.

Magnesium, zinc, and copper: Nuts and seeds provide a range of minerals that are likely to improve brain function, including magnesium and zinc, both of which are crucial nutrients for the normal functioning of the brain. Magnesium also helps reduce tiredness and fatigue, and it's thought that magnesium has a part in regulating receptors found on nerve cells that help memory and literacy. Copper, also found in numerous nuts and seeds, is important for brain development and helps the nervous system function properly.

Iron: Iron plays a part in normal brain function; low iron levels can cause feelings of fatigue and may have a negative impact on brain functions such as concentration, memory, and literacy. Red meat provides readily available iron, but if you don't eat meat, there are a variety of plant foods that provide iron.

Hydration and the brain: Finally, always keep well hydrated. Indeed, mild dehydration can have a negative impact on your memory and brain performance.

Nutrition For Longevity : Eating For A Healthy And Vibrant Life

Good nutrition is a critical part of health and development. According to the World Health Organization(WHO), better nutrition is related to better health at all ages, a lower risk of diseases and longevity.

Nutritional Tips For A Diet

Include protein with every meal: Including some protein with every meal can help balance blood sugar. Some studies suggest advanced-protein diets can be beneficial for type 2 diabetes. Other research indicates that balancing blood sugar can support weight management and cardiovascular health.

Eat oily fish: According to research, omega-3 fatty acids in oily fish are essential for cell signaling, gene expression, and brain and eye development. Some studies indicate that omega-3 fatty acids can reduce the threat of cardiovascular disease. Other research suggests the anti-inflammatory parcels of omega-3 may effectively manage the early stages of degenerative diseases such as Alzheimer's and Parkinson's.

Eat whole grains: The American Heart Association(AHA) recommends people eat whole grains rather than refined grains. Whole grains contain nutrients such as vitamin B, iron, and fiber. These nutrients are essential for body functions that include carrying oxygen in the blood, regulating the immune system, and balancing blood sugar.

The saying 'eat a rainbow' is to help remind people to eat a variety of multicolored fruits and vegetables. Varying the color of plant foods means that someone gets a wide variety of antioxidants beneficial to health.

Eat your greens: Dark,leafy greens are rich in vitamins, minerals, and antioxidants. The Department of Agriculture (USDA) suggests that folate in leafy greens may help protect against cancer, while vitamin K helps with osteoporosis.

Include healthy fats: A person can replace these fats with unsaturated fats, which they can find in foods such as avocado, oily fish, and vegetable oils.

Use extra-virgin olive oil: As part of the Mediterranean diet, extra virgin olive oil has benefits for the heart, blood pressure, and weight, according to a 2018 health report. A person can include extra virgin olive oil in their diet by adding it to salads or vegetables or cooking food at low temperatures.

Eat nuts: According to the AHA, eating one serving of nuts daily in place of red or processed meat, French fries, or deserts may profit health and prevent long-term weight gain. The AHA hints that Brazil nuts, in particular, may help someone feel strong and stabilize their blood sugar. Get enough fiber: According to the AHA, fiber can help improve blood cholesterol levels and lower the risk of heart disease, obesity and type 2 diabetes. People can get enough fiber in their diet by eating whole grains, vegetables, and beans.

Increase plant foods: Research suggests that plant-based diets may help with fat and obesity. According to some studies, including more plant foods in the diet could reduce the threat of developing conditions such as diabetes and cardiovascular disease.

Try beans: Beans are a good source of protein for people on a plant-based diet. Still, those who eat meat can eat it on many meat-free days a week. Beans also contain dietary fiber, vitamins, and minerals.

Nutritive Tips For What To Drink

Drinking plenty of healthy fluids has multitudinous health benefits. Health experts recommend these tips.

Drink water: Drinking enough water every day is good for overall health and can help manage body weight, according to the Centers for Disease Control and Prevention(CDC). Drinking water can prevent dehydration, which can be a particular risk for older adults. Still, they can add some citrus slices and mint leaves to increase the appeal or drink herbal teas if someone doesn't like plain water.

Enjoy coffee: A 2017 study suggests that moderate coffee consumption of 3–5 mugs a day can reduce the risk of type 2 diabetes, Alzheimer's diseases, Parkinson's diseases and cardiovascular diseases. According to the same study,the recommended amount is reduced to 2 mugs per day for pregnant and lactating people.

Drink herbal tea: According to research, catechins in green, black, and other herbal teas may have antimicrobial properties. Herbal teas, such as mint, chamomile, and rooibos, are caffeine-free and help keep someone hydrated throughout the day.

Nutrition Tips For Foods And Drinks To Avoid

It's important to cut back on foods and drinks that may have dangerous health consequences. For instance, a person may want to

Lower sugar intake

According to researchers, dietary sugar, dextrose, and high fructose corn syrup may increase the risk of cardiovascular diseases and metabolic patterns. People should look out for hidden sugars in foods that manufacturers label as names ending in "ose," for example, fructose, sucrose, and glucose. Natural sugars, such as honey and maple syrup, could also contribute to weight gain if someone eats them too frequently.

Drink alcohol in moderation

Dietary Guidelines Americans recommend that if someone consumes alcohol, it should be in moderation. They advise up to one drink per day for ladies and up to two drinks per day for men.Excessive drinking increases the risks of chronic diseases and violence and, over time, can impair short- and long-term cognitive function.

Avoid sugary drinks.

The CDC associates constantly drinking sugary drinks with weight gain and obesity,type 2 diabetes, heart diseases, kidney diseases, tooth decay and cavities,gout, a type of arthritis. People should limit their consumption of sticky drinks and, rather, drink water.

Eat less red and processed meat

A large prospective study in the British Medical Journal Trusted Source indicates that U.S. adults eating more red and processed meat had advanced mortality rates. Actors who shifted meat for other protein sources, such as fish, nuts, and eggs, had a lower risk of death in the eight-time study period.

Avoid processed foods

According to a review in Nutrients, eating ultra-processed foods can increase the risk of numerous diseases, including cancer, irritable bowel syndrome, and depression. People should rather consume whole foods and avoid foods with long lists of processed ingredients.

Other Good Health Habits

There are several ways a person can improve their health in addition to consuming healthy foods and drinks.

Support your microbiome

 A review in Nutrients suggests that a high-quality, balanced diet supports microbial diversity and can impact the risk of chronic diseases. The authors indicate that including vegetables and fiber is dietary to the microbiome. Again, eating too many refined carbohydrates and sugars is detrimental.

Consider a vitamin D supplement

 The recommended dietary allowance for vitamin D is 15 micrograms, or 600 transnational units per day, for adults. A good number of people get part of their vitamin D from the sun and also from some foods. People with darker skin, aged adults, and those who get lower exposure to sun during sunny and winter climates may need to take a vitamin D supplement.

Be aware of portion sizes

 Being mindful of portion sizes can help people take care of their weight and diet.

Use herbs and spices

 A review suggests that the active compounds in ginger may help with oxidative stress and inflammation that occur as part of aging.Curcumin in turmeric is anti-inflammatory and may have defensive effects on health. According to research garlic has numerous benefits, including anti-inflammatory, antimicrobial, and antioxidant properties.

Give your body a rest by fasting

 Intermittent fasting has to do with eating either overnight or on specific days of the week. This may reduce energy input and have health benefits. According to a 2020 review, intermittent fasting may improve blood pressure, cholesterol levels, and heart health.

Keep a food journal

 The American Society for Nutrition says that keeping a food journal can help people track calories, see how important they're eating, and recognize food habits. Keeping a food journal could help you keep track of your weight and eat a more healthy diet.

Wash fruits and vegetables

Raw fruits and vegetables can contain dangerous ingredients that could make someone sick, according to the CDC. Always wash the fresh produce when eating it raw.
Don't microwave oven plastic containers
 Research suggests that microwaving food in plastic holders can release phthalates, which can disrupt hormones. Experts recommend heating food in glass or ceramic holders that are microwave oven-safe.
Eat varied recipes
 Numerous people eat the same recipes regularly. Varying foods and trying different recipes can help someone achieve their needed nutrient input. This can help when choosing to eat a variety of vegetables or protein.
Eat mindfully
 In a 2017 study, mindful eating helped adults with obesity eat smaller sweets and manage their blood glucose.

Concluding remarks

 The power of a diet is like a superhero that energizes your health and well-being. When you eat a balanced diet packed with nutritional foods, you are giving your body the energy and nutrients it needs to serve at its best. It's like giving your body a power boost!. A healthy diet can help with diseases, improve your mood, boost your immune system, and keep your weight in check. Unleash the power of a nutritional diet and energy for a supercharged life. Eating a healthy diet can have a positive impact on your overall well-being. It's all about making smart food choices and nourishing your body with the right nutrients. By incorporating a variety of fruits, vegetables, whole grains, lean proteins, and healthy fats into your diet, you will be giving your body the energy it needs to thrive. Plus, staying hydrated by drinking plenty of water is important too. So keep up the great work and continue to prioritize our health through a balanced diet. Trying different diets and determining what works for you, can be quite an intriguing and informative process. The key is to experiment with colorful eating patterns and pay attention to how your body responds. You could try different diets, consulting with a nutritionist, or even keeping a food journal to track your progress. Remember; it's all about finding a balance that suits your life and makes you feel best. Nutrients are like superheroes for our bodies. They give us the energy we need to stay active and support our immune system to fight off those pesky origins. But that is not all! Nutrients also play a crucial role in keeping our organs healthy and performing properly. They help regulate our heart, brain, liver, and other important organs. Incorporating whole, unprocessed foods into our diet comes with a bunch of benefits! These foods are packed with essential nutrients, fiber, and antioxidants that are naturally present. They provide us with a wide range of vitamins, minerals, and phytochemicals that support our overall health. Let's embrace the power of whole, undressed foods for a healthier and happier life. Be aware that eating practices can have a huge impact on our overall health! When we eat mindfully, we pay attention   to our body's hunger and wholeness cues, as well as the taste, texture, and satisfaction we get from our food. This helps us develop a healthier relationship with food and our bodies. Nutritional food choices have the power to nourish our bodies and enhance our lives in numerous ways. They contribute to better brain function, mood regulation, and overall internal well-being. Nutritional food choices are like the ultimate energy for our bodies. They give us the energy we need to enjoy our day and keep us feeling strong and healthy. Plus, they are packed with all the good stuff like vitamins, minerals, and antioxidants that support our overall well-being. When we make nutritional food choices, we are giving ourselves a best chance to live our lives to fullest

Final Thoughts

Our vulnerable system functions stylishly with a balanced diet that includes a range of vitamins and minerals. Not one

single food or nutrient will help with illness, but incorporating a variety into a balanced diet each day will help boost your body's vulnerable functions and fight infections.Nutrition is an important aspect of health, and people should begin leading a healthy life by making little changes to their diet. It's also important to remember other crucial aspects of health, such as exercise and exertion, stress strategies, and acceptable sleep.

www.ingramcontent.com/pod-product-compliance
Lightning Source LLC
Chambersburg PA
CBHW061017260726

48661CB00005B/2223